Assessing Dyslexia

Assessing Dyslexia guides readers through the design, administration, and interpretation of dyslexia assessments. Grounded in research on the linguistic and neural foundations of dyslexia, as well as the clinical outcomes of reading and writing processes, this concise volume provides a comprehensive framework for assessment, diagnosis, and intervention. Utilizing detailed examples to illustrate methodology and concepts, this book is critical reading for students looking to deepen their understanding of assessment, literacy, and the written language challenge.

Becky Kennedy is former Associate Professor and Humanities Department Chair at Lasell College, USA.

Kathleen Ryan is Associate Professor in the Education Department at Hellenic College, USA.

Assessing Dyslexia

Becky Kennedy and Kathleen Ryan

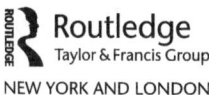
Routledge
Taylor & Francis Group

NEW YORK AND LONDON

First published 2021
by Routledge
52 Vanderbilt Avenue, New York, NY 10017

and by Routledge
2 Park Square, Milton Park, Abingdon, Oxon OX14 4RN

Routledge is an imprint of the Taylor & Francis Group, an informa business

Library of Congress Cataloging-in-Publication Data
A catalog record for this title has been requested

ISBN: 978-0-367-68309-2 (hbk)
ISBN: 978-0-367-68177-7 (pbk)
ISBN: 978-1-003-13685-9 (ebk)

Typeset in Sabon
by Taylor & Francis Books

Contents

Preface

The story of literacy is a chapter in the story of language; it is also a travel story, because literacy allows us to travel to the end of the world and beyond. By not only experiencing our immediate context but also projecting ourselves beyond that context in order to ponder the wide world, we discover new meanings. Written text is conceived on concreteness, but the achievement of literacy opens the door to abstraction: to the unimagined universe.

We enter literacy with complete—and implicit—knowledge of the spoken language upon which written language is constructed. The written form borrows the systems of the spoken form: It utilizes the *lexicon* (the word listings), the *morphology* (the system of word structures), the *syntax* (the system of sentence and phrase structures), and the *semantics* (the system of meaning structures). Written language also references, crucially, the *phonology* (the system of sound structures) of the spoken language, another natural system whose minimal structural unit is the *phoneme*. For efficacy, we produce and apprehend spoken language by *syllables* (minimal rhythmic units) rather than by phonemes; we therefore need not be aware of the abstract phoneme segments in the speech stream. Although the phonology of the spoken language is cognitively opaque to us at the phonemic level, we spend our first year of life mastering the phonemic system of that spoken language; in a few short years, we will have acquired the language's morphology and syntax as well. The rapidity of that acquisition is one of the hallmarks of our evolved and natural capacity to acquire spoken language; another index of its evolved character is its biologically programmed development that unfolds through exposure and transaction rather than by instruction.

Written language differs from the natural spoken language in that it is a constructed entity, a human invention, governed not by natural principles like those of the spoken language but by artificial conventions. And unlike spoken language, whose acquisition is spontaneous and effortless, requiring only a sampling of language data and the social opportunity to interact linguistically, written language is taught. The written language has its own systems that are—unlike the phonology, morphology, syntax, and semantics of the spoken language—created systems. The written language systems are those of *orthography* (the spelling system) and *phonics* (the mapping system whereby *graphemes*—letters or letter clusters that are orthographic units—represent the phonemes of natural language). Most children require instruction to master the reading and spelling of written language; in that instruction, not only the elements of the written language systems—the graphemes and the phonics conventions—but also the segments in the natural language systems that are coded in the written language system must be made explicit. When we speak and listen, we need be no more than implicitly aware of the abstract phoneme. To spell and read, however, we must access and segment the phonemes in words so that the sound–symbol associations in the orthographic code may be applied. The phonemic segmentation must be explicit; the abstraction of the phoneme must be concretized.

The concrete underbody of the written language is reflected not only in the explicitness of its taught and learned conventions but also in the fact that written language is committed to a surface. That surface might be that of a page, or a screen, or a virtual site, but this commitment affords written language a longevity that spoken language, committed to the moment of its occurrence, does not have: At the moment of utterance, the speech imprint is already beginning to vanish. Intrinsically situated in time and in space, spoken discourse is situational; it is wedded to the context of its utterance and relativized to the features of the moment of utterance, as are many of the words of spoken discourse, such as *this, that, yesterday, tonight, left, right, I.* These words shift in significance as the context shifts; they reference aspects of the singular context in which the utterance occurs. A written document, in contrast, traverses time, space, and orientation; it is intended to carry its meaning with it wherever it goes. And here, the abstract potential of written text begins: Written text is an important site and vehicle for abstract thought. Its longevity permits greater complexity than would occur in spoken discourse; by the time we enter the fourth grade, we are reading words, sentences, and texts that are more complicated both in form and in content than those that occur in our spoken discourses. As skilled readers, we flip pages or scroll texts; apprehension of highly complex data and concepts is possible because we can revisit, reread, and review. The decontextualized character of written text and the potential for complexity not only in the message but also in our interior response to it invite us, as readers, to transact with content: to analyze, to synthesize, to abstract.

We see then that the concreteness imperative governs the print code and its first mastery, yet the written text is a site for complex, abstract, and unleashed thought. As we will see, the constraints on the print code on which the second-order, artificial written language system depends may make that first mastery difficult—very difficult, for some learners. Once the door to the world of literacy is unlocked, however, the rewards are immeasurable. And there is a key.

1 The Study of Dyslexia

Dyslexia

> Dyslexia is a specific learning disability that is neurobiological in origin. It is characterized by difficulties with accurate and/or fluent word recognition and by poor spelling and decoding abilities. These difficulties typically result from a deficit in the phonological component of language that is often unexpected in relation to other cognitive abilities and the provision of effective classroom instruction. Secondary consequences may include problems in reading comprehension and reduced reading experience that can impede growth of vocabulary and background knowledge.
>
> (International Dyslexia Association, 2002; see Lyon et al. 2)

Dyslexia, challenge in learning to read, is the most commonly occurring developmental learning challenge and is profound in its effect. The dyslexic child struggles to master reading and writing skills; while peers engage with text, the dyslexic student seeks access to a world of print. We cherish the rewards of that access: the ability to travel beyond spatial and temporal limits through literacy. Reading and writing permit each of us to maintain an interior discourse with the self, as well as a dialogue with those who have preceded, those who will follow, and those who will never be encountered: to bypass the contingencies of time, place, memory, and presence. Through the literacy activities of reading and writing, communities, too, advance to a level of complexity and novelty that would be impossible without the platform of text.

As the capacity to be literate changes the individual and transforms society, the reading brain has also undergone a rearrangement. Neurological circuits designed for other functions have been recruited to accommodate the cultural invention of the print code: In order to engage in the artifice of text creation and recognition, we capitalize on our command of the spoken language we have naturally and spontaneously acquired and on its neurological underpinnings. Speaking and listening are the outcomes of an evolved and innate capacity, and we are pretuned to human speech when we acquire spoken language. Written-language forms are, in contrast, invented; writing is a cultural tool, and we are not prepared neurologically to process written text. As we recode our natural language output in written form, reassembling spoken forms as written text, the complete but implicit knowledge of language structures that we use continuously but subconsciously in spoken expression and communication must be made cognitively visible to us: Our implicit knowledge of language must be made explicit. We apprehend spoken language at a precognitive level; a speaker and listener need not be cognizant of the units of spoken language in order to produce and process speech. On the other hand, the reader who encounters written language and the writer who generates print must utilize those very objects that the speaker and the listener are at liberty to disregard: the minimal segments of spoken language. It is here that dyslexia begins.

The study of dyslexia represents one of the most successful research enterprises on which the modern global intellect has embarked. The findings of educators, clinicians, psychologists, and neurologists have directed researchers toward highly productive agendas that have deepened our understanding of dyslexia's sources and have inspired the development of innovative, effective treatment programs. One characteristic of dyslexia that has fueled efforts to probe its source and refine its treatment is its demographic indifference. Like the great universals of the human condition— faith, death, love, suffering—dyslexia does not select for economic or social class, nor parenting philosophy, nor academic curriculum, nor instructional excellence, nor intelligence quotient, nor spoken-language culture, even though every one of these putative learning factors has a special effect on outcomes for a dyslexic learner. The etiology of dyslexia is neural; situated neurologically, too, are the reading process and the processing of the spoken language on which a writing system is based. Critical in the character of dyslexia, however, is its insularity: The challenged single-word reading and spelling that are the hallmarks of dyslexia need not be accompanied by other types of learning difficulties or by circumstantial challenges. Dyslexia may but need not be accompanied by attention challenge, spoken-language challenge, challenge in text comprehension, curricular disadvantage, or a home dialect that is different from the cultural grapholect—the literacy dialect.

Advances in our understanding of skilled and challenged reading benefit from the productive intercourse of international, intercultural, and interdisciplinary efforts to understand and treat dyslexia. Key insights have been attained regarding the nature of the underlying deficit, its presentation, the pertinent neural underpinnings, and the genetic sources.

Insights from Natural Language

The preceding observations invite a question: If it is the spoken language that the brain, in the presence of minimal spoken-language data in social context, is configured to acquire naturally, whereas the written language is constructed, both in its organization and in its neurological circuits, on components designed on behalf of the spoken form, why would difference in the brain base impede written-language functions without a concomitant disruption of the spoken language? The insight that resolves this question implicates the relation between spoken and written language and illuminates the core challenge in dyslexia.

Written language is founded on spoken language; decades of research indicate that both the achievement of reading and the challenge to reading that appears in dyslexia are understood in terms of aspects of the phonological component of spoken language. The phonological system of language is the sound module; the phonology of a language includes its inventory of distinctive sounds and the sound features that distinguish them, as well as the structural principles that govern their interaction. The minimal sound unit in that phonological system is the phoneme; the phoneme is an abstraction, representing a set of speech sounds that, for native speakers of any language, are perceived as equivalent in sound value. A phoneme may be variously realized on a phonetic (speech sound) level, depending on its phonological context in the speech stream. For instance, in the following sentence, the instances of the phoneme /t/ vary at a phonetic (perceived speech sound) level: *Tim Burton stole a pat of butter from the tray.* Speakers and listeners collapse the distributional variants of /t/ and observe that the phoneme /t/ occurs six times in the sample sentence; phonetic attention reveals, though, that each instance of /t/ in that sentence has a distinctive phonetic realization, conditioned by its local speech context. Crucially, the speaker and the listener need not achieve explicit awareness of those distinctive phones (sounds) in order to issue and process the sentence. Liberman (*Speech*) characterizes the phones of speech as *gestures* rather than sounds. In forming a syllable, the speaker produces a sequence of gestures, each of which is associated with a target phoneme, but those gestures are folded together in syllabic context by an efficiency-driven coarticulation, under which gestures merge and overlap in the service of speed. The listener in turn unpacks that syllable as a sequence of phonemes; the match between speaker intention and listener perception is achieved because both are tuned by a special, automatized speech mode of perception (439).

Speech and writing diverge here: The speaker and the listener need not be aware of the phonemic composition of the syllable or of the word, but the reader and speller must draw on awareness of phonemic segmentation in order to decode and encode print messages. And this difference between speech and writing is critical to an understanding both of the achievement of reading and of the failure of that achievement. Written languages that utilize alphabetic systems are founded on the *alphabetic principle*: Graphic symbols map onto the sounds of spoken language. English *graphemes*—letters and letter clusters—represent the English phonemes. As Liberman observes, reading and writing processes have critical roots in spoken language, yet the two modes of communication divaricate in important ways. Spoken language is biological in its provenance; written language is a cultural artifact. In order to produce or apprehend spoken forms, a speaker and a listener need not be aware of their phonetic structure, because those forms are "the automatic results of a precognitive specialization for phonological communication" (Liberman, *Speech* 444). Acquisition of natural (spoken) language therefore neither requires the segmentation of a syllable as a string of phonemes nor prepares the speaker to master the alphabetic principle. Liberman and Whalen explain that when learning to read, however, "the child must ... learn to put his attention where it never had to be ... Speech does not require phonemic awareness" (193). Spoken and written language differ with respect to the role of the abstract phoneme in language processes; this difference underlies the profound significance of the phoneme's abstract character to the achievement of reading skill and to the failure of that achievement.

Alvin Liberman's groundbreaking work on speech production and perception had its roots in a 1944 project: Liberman was invited by scholars at the Haskins Laboratories in New Haven, Connecticut, to help develop the sound output for a reading machine for the blind. In this instrument, each printed letter would be translated as a distinctive sound that the blind user would associate with a consonant or vowel sound in the language. Scanning print, the machine would pair each alphabet letter with an acoustic pattern that could be learned and recognized by the user. Under the view of speech assumed in this enterprise, which Liberman calls the conventional *horizontal view*, speech is composed of an "acoustic alphabet, with segments of sound as discrete as the letters that convey them" (Liberman, "How Theories of Speech" 4). Under that conventional view, speech comprises a constituent sequence of sounds, perceived by general cognitive/auditory capacities; each sound arrives at phonetic significance via a cognitive translation. In this horizontal model, the listener would understand speech in the same way that print is apprehended, interpreting each sound in sequence—just as, in reading, the letters that constitute a text are interpreted in sequence. In both cases, the units—sounds and letters—would be strung together like beads on a string.

Liberman's project failed, because the temporal resolving power of the human ear was inefficient under these conditions (Liberman, *Speech* 6): The rate of normal speech is ten times the maximal rate at which reading machine users could follow and interpret a translated acoustic pattern sequence. That failure inspired Liberman's lifelong research agenda, as he sought to understand what afforded natural speech its special rate and efficiency. Liberman concluded that speech was not a general auditory signal comprising a sequence of sounds of a general auditory type; under Liberman's unconventional *vertical view*, the phonemes—basic units—of speech are not concrete auditory entities but instead articulatory *gestures* that do not line up as would beads in a necklace but, rather, overlap and merge in efficient articulation of the syllable. This view is termed *vertical* because a vertical view of language is adopted, such that "speech is a constituent of a vertically organized system, specialized from top to bottom for linguistic communication" (Liberman and Whalen 187). From syntax to phonetics, structures and processes are special to language. The speaker's signal codes gestures linguistically; the listener in turn hears speech and resolves the speech signal by recovering the phonemic code of that speech stream.

The language-specific coding and retrieval processes of, respectively, the speaker and the listener permit parity in the expression and reception of that signal. Crucially, however, these processes are precognitive; they are cognitively opaque: "Because the speech specialization is a module, its processes are automatic and insulated from consciousness" (Liberman, *Speech* 442). Before they read, children are aware of words, but neither a speaker nor a listener need be aware of phonemes—of the abstract gestural units of the speech stream—in order to formulate or perceive speech. Articulating an insight that is of critical significance both in educational curriculum design and in an understanding of dyslexia, Liberman reminds us that "phonological awareness, which is necessary for application of the alphabetic principle, does not come for free with mastery of the language" (*Speech* 442). Speaking does not entail awareness of the internal composition of the speech stream; in fact, the qualities of speech that make it most effective for communication obscure further any distinctive reflexes of its abstract units.

Articulation and gestural merger efface recognizable correspondences between the acoustic stimulus—the syllable—and its abstract phonemic constituents. Liberman concludes, "Reading/writing are hard just because speaking/listening are easy" (*Speech* 429). Prioritized by its natural status, "speech is a product of biological evolution," while writing "is a triumph of applied biology" but is, itself, "an artifact" (435). This last insight—that speech is an evolved capacity and writing is an invented tool—accounts for the robustness and effortlessness of spoken-language acquisition but also predicts the wide variation observed in individual reading and spelling achievement trajectories.

The critical distinction between the natural character of spoken language and the artificial nature of written language points us toward the overarching challenge of dyslexia: As Liberman asserts and Shaywitz emphasizes, "The effortless and seamless nature of spoken language has everything to do with why reading is so hard for dyslexic children" (Shaywitz 49). Shaywitz points out that speaking and reading reference the same building block, or "particle": the phoneme, an abstract linguistic sound unit. As Liberman's account of speech processing indicates, the phoneme serves as a codal interface between speech production and speech perception; reference by both parties to that abstract phonemic level permits parity across expression and reception, and the precognitive nature of that reference permits the efficiency that makes speech communicatively meaningful. That cognitive opacity, however, obviates for the speaker a requirement that is fundamental to the reader: phonemic transparency. Written language references the phonology of spoken language as intermediary between the code of text and its content. The speaker encounters speech with an innate preparedness to process it linguistically; the reader, however, is not equipped with a similar innate and precognitive disposition to process text. The speaker is pretuned to the data of speech; the reader is not pretuned to alphabetic data.

Phonemic Awareness and Dyslexia

Liberman's account of the difference between speech and reading illuminates the critical contribution of the young reader's achievement of phonemic awareness in reading development; it also elucidates the special vulnerability of phonemic awareness in dyslexia. Uhry and Clark note the complex relationship between phonemic awareness and reading: Phonemic awareness is "causal" (101) in the mastery of single-word decoding (cf. Bradley and Bryant). The causal relationship between phonemic awareness and decoding achievement, moreover, is bidirectional; decoding growth fosters capacity to analyze the speech stream at the abstract phonemic level. Morais and Mousty argue for this "interactionist position" that "the causes of phonemic awareness are mainly two: linguistic development and alphabetic instruction" (194).

In this regard, Vellutino and Fletcher review the challenges observed in dyslexic readers: They note that operationally, dyslexia in struggling young readers is "manifested in basic and pervasive deficiencies in word identification, phonological (letter-sound) decoding, and spelling" (363): in vitiated response to text, that is, at the single-word level. They remind us that challenged linguistic processing at the sentence and text levels—manifested as reductions in language comprehension, syntactic processing, and vocabulary apprehension—may but need not accompany challenged decoding and encoding of single-word print; crucially, however, single-word decoding competence has been shown (e.g., Hoover and Gough) to be requisite for skilled reading of print: for reading competence. Vellutino and Fletcher point to

> convergent evidence that most children with dyslexia have significant difficulty learning to map alphabetic symbols to sound and acquiring facility in phonological decoding ... Such difficulties, in turn, appear to be related to limitations in their ability to acquire phonological awareness ... [with] evidence for a causal relationship between deficiencies in phonological awareness and alphabetic mapping on the one hand and difficulties in acquiring facility in word identification and spelling on the other.
>
> (Vellutino and Fletcher 364)

This observed causal chain underscores the status of the phonological processing deficit as the core deficit in dyslexia.

Liberman's insight that reading is hard because speech is easy (*Speech* 427) is fundamental: The opacity of the abstract phonemic level of spoken language is due to the precognitive character of speech processing. Abstract phonemic segments code speech but are not consulted for the production and processing of the speech stream; for reasons of efficiency, both speech production and speech processing are automatic and precognitive in their occurrence. Incipient readers are not biologically prepared to segment the sound stream of language into abstract phonemes; many children learn phonemic segmentation, but about one in five children will struggle to segment phonemically. However, phonemic awareness, the "insight that every spoken word can be conceived as a sequence of phonemes" (Adams 15), is critical to the activation, for reading and spelling success, of the alphabetic principle that letters and letter sequences map to phonemes. Children who do not perceive the speech stream as a sequence of abstract phonemic segments will struggle to master the alphabetic principle and will not build a bank of phonics sound–symbol associations; unable to break down or build up a word phonemically, they are challenged by alphabetic reading and spelling.

Confirming the status of phonemic awareness as a critical dyslexia deficit, researchers find that a range of tasks that require phonological processing and alphabet–phoneme mapping challenge dyslexic children: phoneme segmentation, word attack (the decoding of orthographically transparent nonwords), and phonological memory tasks such as nonword repetition and number sequence repetition. Vellutino and Fletcher (364) cite the effectiveness of phonological awareness and alphabetic mapping training in the improvement of reading and spelling outcome skills as another index of the causal relation between underlying phonemic awareness challenge and dyslexic outcome challenges.

Mather and Wendling (138) also note the positive effects of phonemic segmentation training on reading growth; in addition, they highlight the dyslexia-specific character of the phonological processing deficit. For instance, Catts et al. point out that dyslexia and specific language impairment (SLI), which involves atypical development in (especially) the phonological, morphological, and syntactic components of spoken language, are potentially comorbid (co-occurring) conditions, with (statistically significant) overlap in their occurrence, yet dyslexia's characteristic phonological awareness and phonological memory deficits are associated specifically with dyslexia; significant phonological processing deficits are not observed in SLI in the absence of dyslexia. Mather and Wendling emphasize, too, the singularity of the deficit that does occur in dyslexia: the specificity of the phonological processing deficit and the concomitant reading and spelling challenges, which are unexpected in relation to other intellectual performance levels. Thus dyslexic individuals may (but need not) struggle with vocabulary or language comprehension. The specificity of the phonological processing deficit not only in dyslexia but also to dyslexia suggests causality between the deficit and the reading and spelling outcomes in dyslexic individuals (Vellutino and Fletcher 364).

Dyslexia Subtype Analyses

Vellutino and Fletcher join other researchers, too, in evaluating subtyping in dyslexia: The heterogeneity in dyslexic presentations has motivated various subtype classification schemes. Studies of acquired dyslexia—reading skill loss in a mature reader, due to brain insult—have historically yielded a three-subtype analysis; Mather and Wendling review those three subtypes. *Phonological dyslexia* is characterized by successful reading of familiar sight words but challenge in tasks such as nonword decoding that require phonological analysis and alphabetic coding skills; the patient who displays *surface dyslexia* successfully applies phonics associations to decode (orthographically regular) nonwords as well as orthographically transparent words but struggles with orthographically opaque exception words; *deep dyslexia* features challenged nonword reading, special challenge on abstract terms or function words, and errors involving semantic miscue (Mather and Wendling 5–6). Seidenberg identifies the localized lesion sites associated with surface and phonological dyslexia: Patients displaying surface dyslexia symptoms generally show trauma in areas where semantic information is coded (the brain's left temporal lobe or linking sites), and patients with phonological dyslexia presentation have undergone trauma in areas where phonological information is coded (the brain's temporoparietal circuit locations) (192–195). Seidenberg describes deep dyslexia as "a more extreme version of phonological dyslexia" (199).

Dehaene, observing that all writing systems seek a balance between the representation of sound and that of meaning, draws a connection to "two routes for reading" (38), whose disruptions have their respective outcomes in phonological and surface dyslexia presentations. He explains that the phonological route processes regular and/or unfamiliar strings: The reader progresses from letters to pronunciation to meaning. In contrast, the lexical route, utilized to process familiar or irregular words, takes the reader from word forms to meaning to word pronunciation. Neither route alone accounts for all contingencies of print; the mature reader integrates the two operations automatically. The phonological and lexical routes are integrated, too, in the dual-route model of reading (cf., e.g., Coltheart): The sublexical, indirect phonological route depends on associations between phonological and orthographic segments; the lexical route bypasses those phonology–orthography connections, circuiting directly from orthography to the lexicon and thereby to meaning. The distinction between the two classes of acquired dyslexic patients distinguished by lesion locus and clinical presentation informs the dual-route model of reading; that model has in turn been applied to distinguish subtypes in developmental dyslexia. Young readers challenged by, for instance, orthographically regular nonword decoding have been identified by some researchers as phonological dyslexics; young readers who read regular nonwords successfully but struggle to read irregular high-frequency words are termed surface dyslexics.

As another dyslexia subtyping approach, the double-deficit hypothesis represents an enrichment of the core-phonological-deficit view of developmental dyslexia. Acknowledging the centrality of phonemic awareness—the insight that the speech stream can be construed as a string of abstract phonemic units—to reading achievement and the central role of phonological awareness challenge in developmental dyslexia, Wolf et al. propose a second key deficit that also predicts dyslexia: a naming-speed deficit that vitiates effective processing of orthographic patterns. Using rapid automatized naming (RAN) tasks—tasks in which the learner names items in a stimulus series as quickly as possible—to explore the possibility that naming speed represents a second core processing deficit in young dyslexic readers, Wolf et al. tested the hypothesis that phonological awareness and naming speed each add unique variance in dyslexic children's reading task performance.

Wolf and her colleagues identified three groups of dyslexic readers: Readers representing 19 percent of their research sample of severely impaired second- and third-graders revealed a phonological processing deficit but typical naming speed, 15 percent showed a naming-speed deficit without phonological processing impairment, and 60 percent displayed a double deficit in both naming speed and phonological processing of the speech stream. (Six percent of the children were unclassified.) Wolf et al. found that phonological processing measures contributed independently to measured reading outcome skill levels but observed that naming-speed measures accounted for reading performance variance beyond the contribution of phonological processing measures. Reading outcomes considered were word attack level (decoding of orthographically transparent non-words), word identification level (decoding of real words), and reading comprehension; although both naming-speed and phonological processing results contributed independently to outcomes on all three measures, the greater variance in word attack was due to phonological processing performance, and the greater variance in word identification was due to rapid naming performance. Wolf et al. distinguish between the phonemic-analysis demands in the word attack task and the orthographic-pattern recognition and fluency demands of the word identification task; they argue that the phonological processing deficit would more directly impact decoding accuracy, whereas the naming-speed deficit would affect reading fluency (63).

Moves to explore dyslexia subtypes are motivated by observed heterogeneity in dyslexia presentations. In the case of the phonological/surface dyslexia approach, Vellutino and Fletcher (371) point to general research support for the phonological subtype of developmental dyslexia but question the possibility of a stable surface subtype, citing Stanovich et al., who posit that "surface dyslexia may arise from a milder form of phonological deficit than that of the phonological dyslexic, but one conjoined with exceptionally inadequate reading experience" (123). More generally, researchers follow the insight articulated by Shaywitz that "the core problem in dyslexia is phonologic: turning print into sound" (87). Considering the phonological processing/naming-speed deficit distinction, Seidenberg advocates the "phonological umbrella" (176) approach, arguing that "the same underlying phonological deficit can affect either speed or accuracy of reading aloud" (177). The phonological processing deficit, reducing automaticity and efficiency, will impact speed on a timed performance but accuracy on an untimed measure: Both miscues and dysfluency stem, in this view, from a single core deficit.

Dyslexia, Phonological Processing, and Language Diversity

It has also been observed (e.g., Paulesu et al., Caravolas) that developmental dyslexia has differing manifestation patterns when we explore diverse cultural and linguistic contexts. The orthographies—spelling systems—of written languages can be classified along a transparency–opacity spectrum: On this orthographic dimension, those languages with transparent orthographies show regular correspondence between orthographic and phonological units, so that the set of sound–symbol relationships can be applied predictably in decoding. Orthographic transparency may be present in an orthography that represents sounds at the phonemic level, such as Spanish or Italian; it may occur in an orthography that utilizes syllabaries such as those of Japanese. A typical reader with access to the set of sound–symbol relationships associated with a transparent orthography can systematically decode familiar words, unfamiliar words, and nonwords with accuracy.

In contrast, languages such as English and French utilize a deep (or opaque) orthography; in such languages, access to the set of sound–symbol relationships is necessary but not sufficient for accurate decoding of real words. Like any language's orthography, the deep orthography of English represents a code; as is the case for any orthographic encoding, the level of that code is abstract. Transparent orthographies in which every symbol maps to a phoneme in the language work at an abstract level, too, because the phoneme, referenced in the application of the alphabetic principle to reading and spelling, is an abstraction. Under a more complex set of sound–symbol pairings in a language like English, however, orthographic ambiguity occurs; certain word and subword units can be decoded in more than one way. In addition, the complex history of the English language has resulted in an orthographic vocabulary that is particularly broad and diverse, and that diversity in the English lexicon leads to irregularity and exceptionality in certain spellings. Some of those idiosyncratic spellings encode everyday words like *was, the,* and *because*; others represent less common words like *yacht, aisle,* and *pharaoh*. As Dehaene (38) points out, a mix of sound- and meaning-based coding occurs across writing systems; it is the balance between the two that varies by system. The relative opacity of English orthography reflects the coding needs of a language system rich in homophony, in phoneme count, and in linguistic history.

Regular words in English and regular nonwords (designed to conform to English sound–symbol associations, by which they can be unambiguously decoded) can be read and spelled with reliable accuracy when the reader/speller consults the set of orthography–phonology correspondences. English, however, consults another abstract language level in its spelling system, that of the morpheme: the minimal meaning unit. English spelling can be characterized as morphophonemic: Both sound units (phonemes) and meaning units (morphemes) may be coded. When spelling a word like *jumped*, for instance, the speller can apply the alphabetic principle to retrieve symbols (*j, u, m, p*) for the first four phonemes. To complete the spelling by representing the fifth phoneme, however, the speller must look to the morphological level. The fifth phoneme, /t/, is the phonological reflex of the morpheme -*ed*, the English inflectional morpheme signifying past tense. Instead of selecting *t* to represent that final phoneme, as a sound-based encoding would suggest, the speller follows English spelling convention and switches to a meaning-based coding, selecting the final letters, *ed*, to encode the past-tense morpheme directly.

Dehaene goes on to review the observation that the occurrence and the manifestation of dyslexia vary across languages. Considering dyslexic outcomes across languages, Paulesu et al. summarize their findings: Emergent readers working in an orthographically shallow language like Italian are supported by the transparency of the alphabetic code and develop phonological awareness more easily; both typical and dyslexic emergent readers of Italian are better able to achieve accurate decoding, but the dyslexic readers are slower and less fluent. Emergent readers in a reading culture whose language is at the opaque end of the transparency spectrum (e.g., English or French), in contrast, begin by displaying the more familiar behavioral outcomes of dyslexia: vitiated accuracy and fluency. Those qualities gradually dissipate as typical reading develops, but dyslexic readers of English continue to display reductions in both accuracy and fluency. Because dyslexic individuals read English words less quickly and less accurately, whereas dyslexic readers of Italian achieve accuracy but not speed, dyslexia appears to manifest itself differently, cross-linguistically, in writing systems whose orthographies contrast in transparency. Caravolas observes, however, that in spite of different reading outcomes across languages, the occurrence of underlying deficits associated with dyslexia is universal: In the dyslexic groups studied, deficits in phonological awareness, short-term verbal memory, and rapid-naming speed have been observed across language cultures.

Seidenberg distinguishes as well between the behavioral outcome and neurology. Arguing for his "phonological umbrella" (176) view, he argues that a phonological deficit is affecting reading outcome performance for both dysfluent dyslexic readers of a transparent orthography (as in Italian) and inaccurate dyslexic readers of an opaque orthography (as in English): The phonological deficit affects both accuracy and speed in the case of deep orthography and only speed in the case of transparent orthography. In the latter case, the reduction in speed leading to dysfluent reading is a reaction deriving from a phonological impairment. Seidenberg points out that the dyslexic readers of both transparent and opaque (deep) orthographies show a common neurological feature: "atypical activation in a brain region involved in phonological processing" (177). Although dyslexic readers of print in languages of the two types show different behavioral outcomes, the atypical neural source is shared. Reading experience in an orthographically transparent language functions therapeutically, just as does reading practice on English text that has been deliberately constructed for regularity in orthography, with regular words selected to build automaticity through iterated retrieval and application of predictable spelling–pronunciation associations. Quantity of reading is therapeutic; the reading therapist therefore selects that *controlled text*—that regularized English text—to remediate reading in the dyslexic English-speaking student. In contrast, any (reading-age-appropriate) Italian text will, by definition, support the development of reading accuracy in the Italian-speaking dyslexic student.

Neural Sources in Reading and Dyslexia

What are the neurological processes underlying reading and reading impairment? Recent advances in brain imaging and in an understanding of the brain's neural systems for reading have confirmed the neurobiological etiology of dyslexia. Emphasizing that written language is an artifice—an invention—Dehaene examines the neural circuits that serve all written languages, with a special focus on the brain's "letterbox" (65), the visual word form area in the brain's lower left occipitotemporal region—the area where the temporal and occipital lobes of the brain meet. Dehaene characterizes the brain's connections as "bushy" (64), such that various written-language functions activate simultaneously in disparate cortical locations during the reading act. The visual word form area serves as a hub that receives graphemic material and then sends it on to pertinent language-processing cortical sites for phonological (sound) and semantic (meaning) translation. Although this letterbox area parses orthographic (spelling) strings visually, that visual response is triggered by the orthographic identity of the perceived print, as revealed in an indifference to print case and location: The response is characterized by "space and case invariance" (Dehaene 91). As Adams explains, "The visual word form area is indifferent to the size or location or even the fonts or cases of letter strings ... the letters have ceded their shapes to their identities" (7). This specialized invariant response of the visual word form area neurons to orthographic stimuli, as a special adjustment to the conventional features of print, indicates, Dehaene argues, that its function as a hub in the reading circuit is a learned function rather than an innately programmed feature of human vision response.

Reading, Dehaene explains, is not an achievement for which the human brain is prewired: The human brain did not evolve for written-language processes, as it did for those of spoken language. Instead, "reading is a cognitive, social, and cultural activity" (71). Written-language capacity, unlike spoken-language capacity, is therefore not robust and shows great diversity in its individual manifestation. Yet skilled readers use the same cortical spaces; Dehaene observes that across readers, "reading acquisition seems to be a highly constrained process that systematically channels information to the same hot spots in the brain" (75). The "cultural invention" (147) of reading, moreover, utilizes cortical space evolved for other functions. Although reading must utilize preexisting structures, inherent plasticity permits neural reuse, subject to neurological limits. Under Dehaene's "neuronal recycling" (147) approach, "cultural change" (147) in the cortex involves repurposing of neural space in a way that is, nonetheless, constrained by neurobiological architecture and evolved limiting features of the existing neuronal networks. The letterbox area, with its capacity to respond to print and then project the properties of that print specimen for linguistic interpretation in other neural sites, has proved to be a "natural cerebral niche" (149) for written language; written forms worldwide have adapted to fit the letterbox area's constraints and opportunities.

That accommodation of written-language form to available neural structure, moreover, extends beyond the letterbox to its broadcasting activation in the brain. Developing his model of two reading routes (38)—a phonological route for processing regular and/or unfamiliar strings and a lexical route for processing familiar and/or irregular words—that are utilized seamlessly by the skilled reader, Dehaene goes on to describe the neurological correlate of the two routes: The two reading modes select distinct cortical paths. In the reading brain, a dorsal (upper) route derives print's phonological output; a ventral (lower) route bridges orthography and its semantic resolution. Diverse writing systems, moreover, use both routes but favor one or the other, depending on the system's level of orthographic transparency: A transparent orthography such as Italian's system would favor activation of the phonological route for decoding; the more opaque orthographic code of English, in contrast, would weight route choice toward the semantic circuit (118).

Seidenberg explains further the operation of the letterbox or visual word form area in the brain's left occipitotemporal region as a reading "*hub*" (202) that routes orthographic input toward resolution as sound and meaning. Seidenberg, like Dehaene, emphasizes that the phonological and semantic interpretive processes occur across various interconnected cortical structures. Via the ventral or lower route, input passes to a semantic hub, situated in the anterior (front part of the) temporal lobe, where lexical and semantic aspects of meaning stored in diverse cortical structures are integrated. Via the dorsal or upper route, input travels to the supramarginal gyrus (part of the parietal lobe, in the upper back part of the brain), which serves as phonological hub where orthographic information pertinent to phonological translation at the abstract phonemic level is received and interpreted. Reflecting the underlying spoken-language source of written language, the supramarginal gyrus and the immediate cortical regions are also implicated in the phonological interpretation of the speech signal.

The sensitivity of a skilled reader's supramarginal gyrus not only to the speech stream but also to print corroborates the identification of its status as a hub in the reading circuit; in this regard, Seidenberg cites work by Ziegler and Ferrand that attests to the cross-modal effect of orthography on the processing of spoken words. Ziegler and Ferrand (and, later, Ziegler et al.) adduce ways in which mature readers' orthographic learning—their knowledge of word spellings—affects their processing of spoken language as they recognize spoken words. These researchers observed that orthographic *inconsistency*—the existence of alternative spelling options for a phonological segment—significantly affected listener response time on tasks calling for a response to sound properties of target words. (Recall that the deep orthography of English affords alternative possible spellings for certain phonological word shapes; thus, for instance, *beet* could be spelled *beat, biet,* or even *bete.*) Target words with no orthographic alternatives were associated with a performance advantage: Mature readers responded more quickly on tasks involving attention to speech sound properties of the target terms that had no orthographic alternatives, although the tasks were listening tasks. Crucially, a localized cortical deactivation technique (TMS, or transcranial magnetic stimulation) applied to this phonological hub area temporarily suspended the effect, so that (temporarily) the absence of orthographic alternatives had no effect on spoken response speed. These results illustrate the effects of shared cortical space: The supramarginal gyrus and local cortical regions represent a phonological hub serving both spoken and written language.

More broadly, results such as those of Ziegler and his colleagues illustrate the dynamic role of literacy acquisition. The bidirectional relation observed by Morais and Mousty between decoding skill growth and the development of phonemic awareness shows that phonemic awareness—a sensitivity to the sound structure of spoken language—not only is critical to reading achievement but also can be nurtured by reading growth. The findings of Ziegler et al. reveal cortical shaping by the cultural invention of written language, such that older, innately determined cerebral functions are complicated by contingencies—here, orthographic contingencies—of written language. In this case, the functions of the supramarginal gyrus area, part of the innately prewired spoken-language cerebral system that is sensitive to phonological properties of speech stream segments, are reshaped by effects of written-language processing. Written-language forms have accommodated to the available opportunities in preestablished spoken-language circuits; at the same time, the functions of the individual reader's spoken-language cortical circuit areas are modified by skilled written-language practice.

Adams (17–19) traces the maturation of the brain's visual word form area as an individual develops written-language skill. *Lateralization* (whereby specialization for a particular cognitive function appears in one of the two sides of the brain) for spoken-language processes occurs from birth: Via innately wired programming, the left hemisphere acquires automatic spoken-language receptive and expressive functions. It is only as a consequence of several years of learning and of literacy practice, however, that the left hemispheric visual word form area—the letterbox—develops the specialized response to print—the "invariant recognition of letter strings" (Dehaene 207)—that characterizes the area's automatic process in the mature reader. The letterbox first reveals a prospective specialization in an active response to alphabet letters, as letter recognition is mastered by the emerging reader. Fourth-grade students begin to show an automatic lateralized response in the visual word form area to high-frequency words; adolescents engaged fully in literacy practices finally begin to resemble mature readers in fluent letterbox activation responses. Adams points out the distinctiveness of the print-recognition function of the letterbox: "The recognition of spellings that happens with the visual word form area seems to be the only component of the reading process that belongs exclusively to the domain of print as distinct from the domains of language" (8). The visual word form area, though not biologically designed to serve the processing of print, takes on a print-specific function that grows—over years—with the reader's literacy growth and repeated experiences with printed words.

Critical here are the individual reader's practices, and their richness and frequency; it is on these sustained practices that advancement in the reading developmental trajectory depends, and this dependency is the source of the *Matthew effect* (Stanovich). Referencing a parable in the Bible's Gospel of Matthew, Stanovich observes that as reading develops, the growth gap between good readers and challenged readers widens: The rich become richer and the poor become more impoverished. Children who enter literacy training with appropriate assets in phonological processing will respond to instruction by learning and, most important, will be able to amass the reading experience that leads to reading fluency. At the same time, those children whose phonological processing challenges preclude entry into early literacy will not be able to engage in the literacy practice critical to the achievement of fluency and will fall further and further behind their peers. The biblical passage captures the double loss: "For to every one that hath shall be given, and he shall abound: But from him that hath not, that also which he seemeth to have shall be taken away" (Matthew 25:29). The developmental maturation of the brain's reading circuits and of the visual word form area represents a neurological correlate of the educational effect: Adams (18) notes that the maturation of the visual word form area is associated with a child's reading level rather than with chronological age. It is through iterative activations of print–phonology connections during reading that print patterns and phonological patterns develop the firm links underlying fluency, and the brain's reading circuits acquire traction.

Accompanying advances in the cortical mapping of typical reading circuits is progress in the neurological mapping of dyslexia, such that research points to a "neural signature for the phonologic difficulties characterizing dyslexia" (Shaywitz 82). Seidenberg reviews pertinent findings: This neurological signature of dyslexia appears not only in cortical form but also in brain function and development (209). Literacy development in the typical reader is accompanied by a brain lateralization for reading that follows the lateralization for natural language; that typical reader, maturing, reduces activation in the left frontal area that associates orthographic to semantic processing, with a concomitant increase in posterior (back of the brain) orthographic area activity.

The dyslexic reader, however, displays delay and reduced activation, relative to a typical reading peer, in the critical left-hemisphere cortical areas that process phonology and orthography. While these left posterior (back) reading circuit areas are underactivated, moreover, the dyslexic reader displays compensatory hyperactivation in left and right inferior (lower) frontal areas (Seidenberg 210). Shaywitz explains that by adolescence, this frontal overactivation in dyslexic readers has become a pattern that persists in adulthood (81–82): The neural substrate of dyslexia is tenacious. Shaywitz highlights the "pattern of underactivation in the back of the brain" (82) as dyslexia's neural signature; she points out that compensatory use of right and frontal areas in the maturing dyslexic reader is inefficient. As a consequence, the dyslexic reader may achieve accuracy, but fluency remains compromised (84). Shaywitz explains that the underutilization of the left posterior (back) portion of the reading circuit precludes the development of automaticity in the dyslexic reader; the resort to right-hemispheric and frontal processing permits accuracy but does not support speed.

However, Shaywitz injects significant promise: Brain studies following reading intervention targeting phonological processing issues have indicated that the left-hemispheric neural reading systems in dyslexic readers have responded, displaying further development (85–86); as both accuracy and fluency skills have grown and have become established, "brain repair" (86) has also occurred. In a reversal of the Matthew effect, skill growth permits more extensive reading practice, and that practice in turn nurtures further skill growth—and the establishment of typical reading circuitry. Dehaene notes that under remediation, such normalization still accompanies compensation (259); Shaywitz's observation that dyslexic brain difference persists into adulthood supports the insight that dyslexia has a neurobiological base. Clinically and neurologically, dyslexia is rooted in phonological processing challenge, yet the message is one of hope.

The universality of the neurological source of dyslexia is confirmed as Dehaene points to the findings of Paulesu et al., cited earlier in the discussion of differential manifestations of dyslexia, relative to the transparency–opacity spectrum in orthography. Notwithstanding presentation differences attributed to orthography transparency differences in individual languages, Paulesu et al. observe the same left-temporal underactivation— underactivation in the letterbox area—in dyslexic readers across language cultures: Shaywitz's neural signature. Dehaene states that "Paulesu's results thus point to a universal cerebral origin for dyslexia" (244). Across language cultures, underactivation in the brain's letterbox area, precluding the orthography–phonology correspondence crucial to decoding, accompanies and underlies dyslexia.

Genetic Sources of Dyslexia

Brain research confirms the causal connection between neurobiology and the developmental dyslexia outcome; the common neural findings across language cultures suggest a neurological etiology that is constant across variation in dyslexic presentations due to diversity in local orthographies. The relationship, moreover, between dyslexic outcomes and cerebral circuit patterns is—like that between decoding skill growth and the achievement of phonemic awareness—bidirectional: Atypical reading circuitry accompanies the vitiated literacy skills indicating phonological processing deficit, and intervention targeting phonological awareness deficits not only ameliorates reading and spelling performance but also sets the stage for neural rerouting in more typical, more efficient reading circuitry. This bidirectional effect suggests a reciprocity between biology and reading outcomes that is mediated by the reader's phonological processing capacity.

The role of biology extends beyond brain connections to dyslexia; it includes genetic linking. As Seidenberg (161) notes, dyslexia is *polygenic*: No single gene is associated with its appearance. Because reading is not, as is natural language, an evolved capacity but is, rather, a culturally derived practice, literacy acquisition is not a consequence of "genes for reading" (Pennington and Olson 453). Instead, reading development is affected by the genetically determined character of other abilities whose realization is contingent on evolved capacity.

Pennington and Olson review dyslexia's genetic base, pointing out the overall normal distribution of reading performance level and the non-categorical nature of the condition of dyslexia; dyslexic performance falls in the lower end of that normal distribution. They consider data from the extensive study of twins in the Colorado Learning Disabilities Research Twin Study, at the Colorado Learning Disabilities Research Center (CLDRC). To assess the complex of genetic and environmental factors in reading disability outcomes, CLDRC researchers recruited a large sample of learners in twin pairs in which one member showed academically documented reading challenge; in a control cohort of twin pairs, no pair member carried a diagnosis of reading difficulty. Pennington and Olson explain that the twin-study methodology drew on the assumption of normal variable distribution; the guiding insight was that for heritable skills, identical twin pairs would show greater concordance than would fraternal twin pairs, when genetic contributions to skilled reading and to dyslexia were investigated. Early results revealed dyslexia concordance rate of 70 percent in identical twin pairs but only 48 percent in fraternal twin pairs, a strong index of the heritability of dyslexia (DeFries et al.). In addition to comparing reading outcomes such as single-word identification and spelling, researchers considered component skills such as phonological decoding (nonword reading) and orthographic coding in the twin pairs. A number of pertinent measures showed significance; although deficits in orthographic coding, phonological decoding, phonological awareness, and word reading appeared to be highly heritable, the highest correlation in skill-pair contributions (suggesting a shared genetic influence) was between phonological decoding and word reading. The high correlation between phonemic awareness and phonological decoding, moreover, was not matched in the case of phonemic awareness and orthographic coding, suggesting that it is phonological decoding (rather than orthographic coding) that mediates the genetic effects of phonemic awareness on the skilled reading/dyslexic outcomes (Pennington and Olson).

Pennington and Olson note the key results of genetic research: confirmation of the familial and heritable properties of dyslexia, and mapping of risk gene loci on certain chromosomes (such as 6 and 15). Important, too, is the affirmation of the essential role of phonemic awareness, with phonological decoding serving as the skill bridge in accounting for the dyslexic deficit. Genetic study results support a unified conception of dyslexia and of the core base in impaired phonological processing, which, by virtue of its association with impaired phonological decoding, inhibits single-word reading and spelling.

The Study of Dyslexia

The terrain of dyslexia research includes the etiology and the form of written-language challenge. Illuminating the nature of that challenge is the character of the interface between spoken and written language; from both a linguistic and a neurological perspective, the spoken language serves as substrate to written language. In spite of parallels, interactions, and collusions between spoken and written language, the two language modalities contrast in character. Spoken language represents a natural capacity; we are prewired to acquire and to utilize speech. (Note here that observations about the natural status of spoken language apply fully to signed language; the auditory–vocal channel is not the exclusive modality for natural language, and the innate human language capacity does not depend on speech and hearing for its realization. Sign languages such as American Sign Language—ASL—are formal and complete natural language systems.) Written language, in contrast, is a beautiful invention; we have no innate preparedness for the processing of written text. The second-order character of written language extends to neurology: Reading utilizes preexisting neural structures designed for spoken-language communication and repurposed to process written text. Spoken language, as a natural and evolved capacity, is robust; written-language skill, as a cultural acquisition, is vulnerable, and learners are vulnerable to reading challenge: to dyslexia.

Research findings converge in the identification of a core phonological processing deficit underlying the dyslexic outcome. Because spoken language is apprehended at a precognitive level, neither the speaker nor the listener need attend to the minimal sound units of language. The reader and the speller, however, must be able to segment the speech stream into minimal phonological units—phonemes—in order to apply the sound–symbol pairings on which our alphabetic writing system relies. Learners who are challenged by that segmentation requirement—children who struggle with phonemic awareness—are vulnerable to reading and spelling impairment. With respect to the neurological substrate for successful reading, written-language formats utilize neural architecture designed for spoken language. Like successful reading skill, dyslexic processing displays its characteristic mode in the brain; it also has a characteristic developmental trajectory. Characteristic, too, is a liability: the Matthew effect in reading development, under which children who show a phonemic awareness deficit as they encounter literacy instruction will fall further behind their peers at each stage in reading development. This effect registers the dynamic interaction between underlying assets and deficits, on the one hand, and written-language performance outcomes, on the other. Of great significance, however, is the reversible character of such a dynamic. Identification of the challenge of dyslexia is the first step toward its reversal; the assessment of dyslexia follows.

Works Cited

Adams, Marilyn Jager. "The Relation Between Alphabetic Basics, Word Recognition, and Reading." *What Research Has to Say About Reading Instruction.* Eds. S. Jay Samuels and Alan E. Farstrup. Newark, DE: International Reading Association, 2011. 4–24.

Bradley, Lynette, and Peter E. Bryant. "Categorizing Sounds and Learning to Read: A Causal Connection." *Nature* 301 (February 1983): 419–421.

Caravolas, Markéta. "The Nature and Causes of Dyslexia in Different Languages." *The Science of Reading: A Handbook.* Eds. Margaret J. Snowling and Charles Hulme. Oxford: Blackwell Publishing, 2009. 336–355.

Catts, Hugh W., Suzanne M. Adlof, Tiffany P. Hogan, and Susan Ellis Weismer. "Are Specific Language Impairment and Dyslexia Distinct Disorders?" *Journal of Speech, Language, and Hearing Research* 48:6 (December 2005): 1378–1396.

Coltheart, Max. "Modeling Reading: The Dual-Route Approach." *The Science of Reading: A Handbook.* Eds. Margaret J. Snowling and Charles Hulme. Oxford: Blackwell Publishing, 2009. 6–23.

DeFries, John, Richard Olson, Bruce Pennington, and Shelly Smith. "Colorado Reading Project: An Update." *The Reading Brain: The Biological Basis of Dyslexia.* Eds. Drake Duane and David Gray. Parkton, MD: York Press, 1991. 53–87.

Dehaene, Stanislas. *Reading in the Brain.* New York: Penguin, 2009.

Hoover, Wesley A., and Philip B. Gough. "The Simple View of Reading." *Reading and Writing: An Interdisciplinary Journal* 2 (1990): 127–160.

Liberman, Alvin. "How Theories of Speech Affect Research in Reading and Writing." *Foundations of Reading Acquisition and Dyslexia.* Ed. Benita Blachman. Mahwah, NJ: Lawrence Erlbaum Associates, 1997. 3–19.

Liberman, Alvin. *Speech: A Special Code.* Cambridge, MA: MIT Press, 1996.

Liberman, Alvin, and Doug H. Whalen. "On the Relation of Speech to Language." *Trends in Cognitive Science* 4:5 (May 2000): 187–196.

Lyon, G. Reid, Sally E. Shaywitz, and Bennett A. Shaywitz. "A Definition of Dyslexia." *Annals of Dyslexia* 53:1 (2003): 1–14.

Mather, Nancy, and Barbara J. Wendling. *Essentials of Dyslexia Assessment and Intervention.* Hoboken, NJ: John Wiley & Sons, 2012.

Morais, José, and Philippe Mousty. "The Causes of Phonemic Awareness." *Analytic Approaches to Human Cognition.* Eds. Jesus Alegria, Daniel Holender, José Junça de Morais, and Monique Radeau. Amsterdam: Elsevier Science Publishers, 1992. 193–212.

Paulesu, E., J.-F. Démonet, F. Fazio, E. McCrory, V. Chanoine, N. Brunswick, S.F. Cappa, G. Cossu, M. Habib, C.D. Frith, and U. Frith. "Dyslexia: Cultural Diversity and Biological Unity." *Science* 291 (2001): 2165–2167.

Pennington, Bruce F., and Richard K. Olson. "Genetics of Dyslexia." *The Science of Reading: A Handbook.* Eds. Margaret J. Snowling and Charles Hulme. Oxford: Blackwell Publishing, 2009. 453–472.

Seidenberg, Mark. *Language at the Speed of Sight.* New York: Basic Books, 2017.

Shaywitz, Sally. *Overcoming Dyslexia.* New York: Vintage Books, 2005.

Stanovich, Keith. "Matthew Effects in Reading: Some Consequences of Individual Differences in the Acquisition of Literacy." *Reading Research Quarterly* 21:4 (Fall 1986): 360–407.

Stanovich, Keith E., Linda S. Siegel, and Alexandra Gottardo. "Converging Evidence for Phonological and Surface Subtype Reading Disability." *Journal of Educational Psychology* 89:1 (1997): 114–127.

Uhry, Joanna, and Diana Clark. *Dyslexia: Theory and Practice of Instruction.* Austin, TX: Pro-Ed, 2004.

Vellutino, Frank R., and Jack M. Fletcher. "Developmental Dyslexia." *The Science of Reading: A Handbook.* Eds. Margaret J. Snowling and Charles Hulme. Oxford: Blackwell Publishing, 2009. 362–378.

Wolf, Maryanne, Alyssa Goldberg O'Rourke, Calvin Gidney, Maureen Lovett, Paul Cirino, and Robin Morris. "The Second Deficit: An Investigation of the Independence of Phonological and Naming-Speed Deficits in Developmental Dyslexia." *Reading and Writing: An Interdisciplinary Journal* 15 (2002): 43–72.

Ziegler, Johannes, and Ludovic Ferrand. "Orthography Shapes the Perception of Speech: The Consistency Effect in Auditory Word Recognition." *Psychonomic Bulletin & Review* 5 (1998): 683–689.

Ziegler, Johannes, Ludovic Ferrand, and Marie Montant. "Visual Phonology: The Effects of Orthographic Consistency on Different Auditory Word Recognition Tasks." *Memory and Cognition* 32:5 (2004): 732–741.

2   The Written-Language Evaluation

The Assessment of Dyslexia: The Simple View of Reading

Foundational to an understanding of dyslexia have been insights into the relationship between written language and spoken language. The close relationship between the two language modes, such that the written mode borrows not only the linguistic but also the neural forms designed for the spoken mode, accompanies an essential difference: Spoken language is a natural language system, whereas written language is constructed. As a natural form, a first spoken—or signed—language is not taught; instead, it is acquired in the context of natural development. Children exposed to a sampling of spoken language (or of signed language, in the case of similarly natural sign language acquisition) arrive at the structural principles and assemble the systems not through instruction but in social transactions with caregivers. On the other hand, children are instructed in the conventions of written language. Spoken-language acquisition is spontaneous because children are neurologically prewired to speak; inattentive to its structural elements, because they need not attend consciously to structural segments like the phoneme, children acquire language without effort. Efficiency-motivated coarticulation obscures the segmentation of language in speech context, and that is a good thing for spoken discourse but a liability for the new reader, who must attend to phonemes. Phonemic awareness is nonetheless available to some young learners and can be attained by others in the course of curricular training. For one in five children, though, phonemic awareness is elusive. Such children, who struggle to begin to read because they struggle to abstract phonemic segments in the speech stream, are dyslexic.

Research suggests that the phonemic awareness challenge observed in dyslexic children can be attributed to a core phonological processing deficit; the effects of that deficit are both profound and circumscribed. The deep repercussions include those of the Matthew effect in reading growth (Stanovich), which is a consequence of the transactional relationship between phonological processing skill and reading achievement. The bidirectional nature of that relationship, however, also suggests promise; bidirectional effects and incumbent promise, moreover, are observed at the neural level.

Findings regarding dyslexia's heritability and its polygenetic etiology, likewise, point to its persistence at the genetic level and in the individual lifespan; at the same time, such findings argue for the urgency of identification and treatment. And in the clinical arena—in individual assessment and intervention—the great rewards reside.

The persistence of dyslexia's challenge over the lifespan, consistent with dyslexia's evidence at the genetic level, is criterial in the definition of dyslexia. Equally important is the specificity of dyslexia's challenge, such that literacy underachievement is unexpected in the context of the individual learning profile. Working under the model of the *simple view of reading* (cf., e.g., Gough and Tunmer, Hoover and Gough), Tunmer and Greaney define dyslexia by identifying four parts to dyslexia's definition: "(a) persistent literacy learning difficulties (b) in otherwise typically developing children (c) despite exposure to high quality, evidence-based instruction and intervention, (d) due to an impairment in the phonological processing skills required to learn to read and write" (239). Under the simple view of reading, reading competence (R) is seen as the product of decoding competence (D) and comprehension competence (C): $R = D \times C$. Each of the two factors—decoding competence and comprehension competence—is necessary to and is, alone, insufficient for successful reading; a student requires adequate skill levels in both areas to read text.

An account of reading challenge follows from this view of reading: Proximal sources of reading challenge are written-language decoding and/or linguistic comprehension issues. The model also offers an initial framework for an assessment agenda: If a reading skill reduction has been documented, consider each factor in the model. The product R, that is, can be assessed in an observation of the reader's response to text; the respective factorial contributions to that measured product can in turn be evaluated by measuring D and C: "The simple view clearly asserts that reading ability should be predictable from a measure of decoding ability (e.g., the ability to pronounce pseudowords) and a measure of *listening* comprehension" (Gough and Tunmer 7). Gough and Tunmer go on to draw a connection between reading ability and reading disability, under the simple model: "Perhaps the more interesting implication of the simple view ... concerns reading *disability*" (7). Gough and Tunmer observe that reading ability requires adequate skill in both decoding and comprehension; absence of adequate skill in one or both areas produces reading disability in one of three forms (7). The skill imbalance in which adequate linguistic comprehension accompanies inadequate decoding assets is associated with dyslexia; a "garden variety reading disability" is the consequence of deficits in both decoding and comprehension (8). As the third form of reading disability, Gough and Tunmer adduce *hyperlexia*. More generally, hyperlexia is a reading outcome featuring superior, precocious decoding accompanying comprehension that may be adequate or may be in deficit (cf. Kennedy, Treffert). In the latter case, hyperlexia reverses the dyslexia imbalance, such that a decoding superiority accompanies comprehension challenge. It is in that case of elevated decoding paired with a comprehension deficit that the product—overall reading competence—is reduced.

Reading is a multilevel activity; under the simple view of reading, successful reading can be seen as the product of competence in the two discrete areas of decoding and linguistic comprehension. The complex reading process, however, subsumes diverse behaviors; some pertain to comprehension, and others are associated with decoding. No single skill performance will define a reader's success; instead, an individual's reading behaviors can be understood as an individual profile of balances: of strengths and challenges. In order to understand that profile in the individual reader, we can examine its contours, measuring those challenges and strengths in order to understand how they interact in the literacy domain. We can determine assets on which the reader draws; we can also identify areas of reading breakdown. We observe and measure overt *outcome skills*: outcomes of written-language instruction that addresses single-word decoding and spelling as well as text-level fluency, comprehension, and composition. These conventional written-language behaviors are outcomes of appropriate and effective academic instruction; their growth is contingent, though, on the sufficiency of underlying *component skills* in areas crucial to the development of outcome competencies. Preeminent among component skills is phonological processing capacity, which is a core asset underlying a successful reading outcome and represents the core deficit in dyslexia.

The Emergence of Reading

Outcome skill levels reflect the degree to which a learner is profiting from instruction in the conventions of written language. To examine the various outcome skills associated with reading, we can observe the emergence of reading in the typical learner, noting that in the progression of reading phases, emphases change, yet fundamental concerns remain constant. We note the progressive refinement of phonological sensitivity, the development of alphabetic analysis skill, the persistent expansion of automatic sight recognition, the fluent and flexible application of sound–symbol knowledge, the growth of effective and efficient orthographic processing, and the acceleration of fluent reading and comprehension of connected text.

Chall describes the emergence of reading. During the *prereading stage* (birth to age six), young learners amass knowledge about the world of literacy: about books, about language, and about print. As their mastery of the spoken language matures, they also see that spoken language can be viewed *metalinguistically* (13). The *metalinguistic* insight is the insight that we can reflect on, analyze, and play with linguistic objects such as words, syllables, and phonemes. When children compare, break down, or reconstruct words and word parts—by rhyming words or segmenting them, for instance, into syllables or phonemes—they are developing their awareness of the phonological structure of spoken language that represents the foundation on which written language is constructed. During this stage, children may engage in *pseudoreading*, reciting a story they have listened to; the derivation of meaning from print is a *top-down* process, in that young learners superimpose their own ideas when constructing the text (33).

In the first formal reading stage, the *initial reading and decoding stage*, six- and seven-year-old learners are introduced to the detail of the relationships between spoken and written forms and to the systems of the written language: the orthographic code and the conventions of phonics. Mastering the letters of the alphabet and the sounds those letters represent, those learners build a repertoire of sound–symbol associations that can be applied in encoding and decoding words (Chall 15–16): Children are "glued to the print ... in order to leave the print" (18). Print meanings are derived now in a *bottom-up* process; children obtain textual meaning from the print itself (33). And critical to the mastery of foundational written-language skills during this stage is the phonemic insight—the awareness of the phonemic structure of the spoken language—that must be activated in the application of grapheme–phoneme correspondences to reading and spelling tasks. Chall's second formal reading stage is the stage of *confirmation and fluency*. Seven- and eight-year-old learners address the more complex phonics associations; decoding strategies become established and automatic, and recognition of orthographic regularities and print chunks facilitates the development of fluency that will permit readers to turn their attention to content (18–20).

Looking closely at these early reading stages, Ehri distinguishes the growth of decoding strategy for unfamiliar words and the achievement of automaticity in recognizing familiar words; she examines the development of the automaticity that permits the skilled reader to delegate limited attentional resources to the derivation of meaning from print. Under her approach, the goal in the development of that automatic response to text is the reading of *sight* words; here, she is referring not to the reading of irregular or high-frequency words that must be recognized by sight but to the immediate and effortless recognition of familiar words as single units; this *unitization*, under which words are read as units, supports the fluency that enables the reader to dedicate full attention to comprehension (169).

Ehri distinguishes word recognition and apprehension of meaning in successful reading, recalling the simple view of reading and its formula: $R = D \times C$. Under her analysis, children form connections between written spellings and lexical listings that specify pronunciation and meaning; formation of those connections is mediated, crucially, by alphabetic coding. In order to establish fully automatized access to those connections, the reader of English must master the alphabetic principle, under which phonemes are represented by graphemes: letters or letter clusters. Analyzing text alphabetically and the speech stream phonologically, the reader consults the set of sound–symbol relationships representing the alphabetic code for English. Recoding text phonologically, the reader decodes unfamiliar words; it is at this point that sight-word learning begins, through a *"connection-forming* process. Connections are formed that link spellings of written words to their pronunciations and meanings in memory" (Ehri 170). An orthographic representation and a phonological pattern are both associated with a lexical entry; the alphabetic code connects the two:

> When readers learn a sight word, they look at the spelling, they pronounce the word, they distinguish separate phonemes in the pronunciation, and they recognize how the graphemes match up to phonemes in the word. Reading the word a few times secures its connections in memory.
>
> (Ehri 170)

Each time the reader encounters the word, the memory connection of its orthographic form is affixed to its associated phonological pattern and meaning.

As reading experience accrues, patterning at another textual level becomes apparent to the reader and gains prominence in instruction: Orthographic systematicity becomes a powerful learning support and pedagogic tool. Pertinent orthographic chunks include the orthographic strings representing bound morphemes (e.g., prefixes and suffixes such as *pre-*, *-ing*, or *-tion*) or those representing free morphemes that appear both alone and in compound structures (e.g., *book*, appearing in compounds like *notebook, bookworm, bookmark*, or *pocketbook*). Ehri observes, "As readers learn about spelling patterns that recur in different words, these larger units are used to form connections to remember words" (172). Expertise in the alphabetic system, orthographic awareness (awareness of spelling patterns), and phonological awareness support the achievement of effective and efficient sight-word reading. Ehri explains, "Sight word learning this rapid and lasting is possible only because readers possess a powerful mnemonic system in the form of alphabetic knowledge that is activated when words are read" (172), emphasizing the crucial role of alphabetic knowledge and coding.

Emphasizing the critical role of the reader's effective application of the alphabetic code in the achievement of automaticity, Ehri distinguishes the successive phases in sight-word reading development by the reader's level of alphabetic competency: *prealphabetic, partial alphabetic, full alphabetic*, and *consolidated alphabetic* (173). Children in the prealphabetic phase are not yet familiar with the alphabetic system and therefore do not consult the alphabetic code when recognizing a word. Advancement to the partial alphabetic phase accompanies new learning: Children have begun to learn letter names and/or associated sounds. Because this learning is not yet complete and, crucially, because phonemic segmentation of the word unit has not been fully mastered, the alphabetic code is inconsistently consulted when an unfamiliar word is encountered. Segmentation of initial and final consonant sounds in words typically precedes the identification of interior phonemic segments; sound associations for initial and final consonant letters may therefore be utilized during the partial alphabetic phase.

Facility at alphabet letter recognition, mastery of phonemic segmentation, and access to a full set of sound–symbol relationships are critical to advancement to the full alphabetic phase of reading: These achievements permit readers to arrive at automatic single-word (sight-word) reading: "Children become full alphabetic phase readers when they can learn sight words by forming complete connections between letters in spellings and phonemes in pronunciations" (Ehri 174). Spellings become instances of more general and complete graphophonemic knowledge—knowledge, that is, of sound–symbol relations. When the application of sound–symbol relations is consistent and complete, a word's spelling can become "bonded" in memory to its pronunciation (174). This bonding permits memory retention of a word as a single unit; the achievement of unitization supports the automatic retrieval of the word's pronunciation in response to its orthographic presentation and signals sight-word reading. And as a personal bank of sight words expands, the reader responds to larger orthographic units as well: to spelling patterns for common prefixes, suffixes, and roots, for instance. This latter development accompanies the emergence of the consolidated alphabetic phase. That last advance, which features fluency, highlights the critical status of the achievement of automaticity. Crucially, phonemic awareness, alphabetic knowledge, and secure knowledge of phoneme–grapheme associations have facilitated that achievement.

Comprehension Development

The simple view of reading and its formula—$R = D \times C$—suggest the synchrony of assets in the mature reader, who must achieve proficiency in decoding and coincident competency in comprehension in order to practice skilled reading. We see, however, that the emergence of sophistication in the two areas is typically asynchronous: An early focus on decoding shifts to a later emphasis on—and freeing of attentional resources for—comprehension growth. Comprehension develops at both the single-word level and the textual level. At the single-word level, comprehension skill is reflected in the sophistication of the individual lexicon: the depth and breadth of the reader's vocabulary knowledge.

In his discussion of the Matthew effect, Stanovich adduces the interactions between reading growth and phonological awareness as interactions involving "reciprocal causation" (363); he also highlights the reciprocal transaction between reading growth and vocabulary development. Stanovich explains the special significance of phonological awareness for the earlier achievement of decoding skill (363–364) and points to the compromise in reading development—the "causal chain of escalating negative side effects" (364)—when phonological awareness competency is reduced, observing that "soon after experiencing greater difficulty in breaking the spelling-to-sound code, poorer readers begin to be exposed to less text than their peers" (364). At the single-word level, automaticity growth is compromised, and "slow, capacity-draining word-recognition processes require cognitive resources that should be allocated to higher-level processes of text integration and comprehension" (364). Stanovich points out that the typically advancing reader, in contrast, approaches a competency level at which it is not decoding skill but, instead, more general linguistic skill that is the crucial determinant of reading level (364). Here, reading experience assumes great importance, due to the reciprocal interaction between reading practice and language-cognitive skill status. And it is at this point that the dimensions of the individual lexicon are important, and the bidirectional relationship between vocabulary growth and reading maturation assumes prominence. Vocabulary knowledge, like phonological awareness, shares a bidirectional relationship with reading development: At the single-word level, vocabulary knowledge may be either a beneficiary or a casualty of reading skill. Stanovich observes the strong correlation between reading ability and vocabulary knowledge as reading competency matures (379–380); lexical strength profits from and supports decoding facility and reading growth at the level of the text.

At the textual level, reading comprehension, like decoding mastery and sight-word automaticity, unfolds during the years of its maturation in the typical reader. Chall addresses the refinement of the shift in focus from fluent decoding to comprehension of content—the maturation of textual comprehension as readers advance from learning to read to reading to learn (20). Chall identifies the decoding stage as a first stage in reading development and the confirmation stage as a second stage. During Chall's third stage, that of *reading for learning the new*, fourth-grade students begin to read in order to acquire knowledge. Automatic recognition of word units and fluent processing of text free the reader to focus on text content and to return, in part, to a top-down processing style (33). Students bring their own background knowledge, awareness of diverse text structures, and cognitive schema to bear on a text that now is linguistically more sophisticated than the spoken-language discourses they hear or produce (21), although textual complexity is restricted to a single perspective (22). At the high-school level, however, learners enter Chall's fourth stage, that of *multiple viewpoints*; they read in order to understand different points of view. Building on knowledge gained through earlier reading experiences, high-school readers utilize text to explore ideas more broadly and deeply. Greater cognitive flexibility entails both the acknowledgment of diverse viewpoints and the awareness that linguistic meaning can be construed at multiple levels (23). Meaning might be present explicitly or might be implied; high-school-level reading texts invoke inferential understanding as well as literal comprehension. The demands of still greater complexity and depth characterize written text at the fifth stage, that of *construction and reconstruction*. At and beyond the college level, text comprehension is characterized by active synthesis of material, integrative and critical analysis across bodies of knowledge, and novel thought (24).

Outcome Skills

The simple view of reading suggests those reading outcome areas to be addressed in a written-language assessment. We can also distinguish *outcome skills* and *component skills*. An evaluation of a developing reader's written-language *outcome skills* includes the measurement of achievement in the domains associated with the two factors in successful reading: decoding and comprehension. At the same time, the developmental trajectory of the fluent reader features shows the emergence and maturation of those *component skills* that underlie the achievement of outcome skills. For instance, accurate decoding requires facility in alphabet letter recognition, mastery of phonemic segmentation, and knowledge of the alphabetic code that associates letters and phonemic segments; fluent reading is supported by automatic recognition of orthographic strings as word and subword units. Critical component skill areas are those of phonological processing, automaticity, and orthographic processing. Linking outcome skills and component skills is the Matthew effect: In analogy to the spiritual wealth that accrues, as suggested in the biblical parable, in those who are rich in faith, outcome skill assets increase in learners who begin reading instruction with component skill assets, under Stanovich's literacy account. The outcome skill achievement gap between readers who began with component skill assets and those who did not, moreover, will widen exponentially during the learning years.

What are the measurable reading outcome skills? Ehri underscores the significance of alphabetic competency as readers advance through early reading modes: Advancement from a prealphabetic stance to a partial alphabetic stance requires incipient knowledge of letter names and/or associated sounds. Alphabet knowledge and phonics knowledge—knowledge of sound–symbol associations—represent convention systems that must be consulted in successful early written-language behaviors. Although English orthography is deep, is morphophonemic rather than transparently phonetic, and is multilayered, most English words have regular orthographic shapes; successful reading and spelling require thorough knowledge of regular English sound–symbol correspondences. *Word attack* skill, the ability to apply phonics knowledge to decoding, appears at Ehri's full alphabetic phase and is often measured in nonword reading: The reader decodes a set of invented words, orthographic forms that can be translated unambiguously into phonological forms when sound–symbol association conventions are applied. The phonics application that permits successful nonword decoding also contributes to automatic real-word identification proficiency. *Word identification* skill is supported by secure phonics knowledge, which facilitates the bonding of a word's orthographic shape to its phonological form, so that its pronunciation can be retrieved automatically when the printed word is perceived.

Pertinent skills at the single-word level also include *spelling*. A sensitive index of written-language mastery, spelling can also be an important signal of written-language challenge and is often, in the case of dyslexia, the last area to respond to remediation (Shaywitz 114); Cassar et al. note that "dyslexics' spelling problems are often more severe and persistent than their reading problems" (28). Spelling requires full accuracy; an accurate spelling of a word cannot be derived through partial knowledge. Even with full phonics knowledge, moreover, the translation of sound to print in a spelling—even a regular spelling that follows phonics conventions—is less predictable than is the translation of print to sound. As mentioned in Chapter 1, phonics correspondences yield a single pronunciation for the orthographic string *beet*, for instance; that pronunciation, however, could be spelled *beat*, *bete*, or *biet*, under the application of familiar phonics sound–symbol associations. Awareness of and sensitivity to orthographic patterns of English and increasing familiarity with English orthographic conventions help the speller distinguish the correct spelling of a word from possible yet incorrect spellings, as does word-specific orthographic knowledge; this orthographic sensitivity is achieved during Ehri's consolidated alphabetic reading phase.

The single-word outcome skills of word attack and word identification reflect achievement in *decoding*, the first factor in the simple view of reading equation; because of the close relation of encoding to decoding, performance in the outcome area of spelling also serves as a gauge of a learner's mastery of the alphabetic code and its application in literacy practices. The second factor, *comprehension*, represents language comprehension under the simple reading model. Comprehension plays its critical role at both the single-word and the textual level; at the single-word level, comprehension can be examined in *vocabulary knowledge*. At the textual level, comprehension is displayed as the reader addresses connected text and can be observed through *oral reading of connected text, reading comprehension* measures, and *listening comprehension* responses, with listening comprehension the more apt measure of the linguistic comprehension referenced in the simple view of reading.

Oral reading of connected text, reading comprehension performance, and listening comprehension performance offer different windows into overall language comprehension. Oral reading of connected text also provides insight into decoding skill, insofar as oral reading fluency is a function of both rate and accuracy of decoding; each word in the text string must be retrieved accurately and automatically in order for the reader to move fluently through sentences and paragraphs. Fluent reading of connected text differs, however, from the fluent reading of a word list: Fluent reading of text is informed by apprehended content. That apprehension is reflected in the oral reader's prosody—the use of intonation, pitch, and rhythm in ways that respect larger syntactic units such as phrases and clauses and reflect semantic and pragmatic import in the content. Prosody and expressive style reflect awareness of language structures at the phrasal and sentence levels; these oral reading features reflect, too, the reader's sensitivity to broader aspects of the text—to the reader's understanding of the text as meaningful and coherent. Performance on reading comprehension probes may be affected, to varying degrees, by decoding competence; to observe language comprehension in a reading assessment without the possible confound of decoding challenge, measurement of listening comprehension is important.

Comprehension can therefore be assessed at different levels and in different modalities. At the single-word level, we are interested in the dimensions of a reader's lexicon—its depth and breadth—and in the reader's understanding of lexical denotation and connotation both for decontextualized terms and for words in context. At the textual level, content recall is of interest; we look not only for the retrieval of text details but also for an account that indicates grasp of overall textual structure and purpose. We consider, likewise, responses to content questions that indicate inferential as well as literal comprehension of text material. In addition, we can utilize both reading and listening modalities to measure the comprehension of written text. Reading comprehension measures permit the observation of the quality of comprehension of a text read orally or silently. Listening comprehension measures reveal the learner's capacity to extract meaning from text presented orally; the learner listens to a text rather than reading it and then responds to the same types of text-based probes that would be administered under a reading comprehension assessment. Utilizing the listening modality, we have an opportunity to observe comprehension unconstrained by the demands of decoding,

Measurement of text comprehension in a listening modality is especially important when a diagnosis of dyslexia is either present or possible, because the presence of dyslexia can limit reading comprehension. The dyslexic reader's vitiated decoding may reduce access to content; in addition, challenged decoding may consume attentional resources needed for full comprehension. Oral presentation of text for comprehension assessment in the listening modality obviates both constraints on comprehension performance and permits the observation of comprehension unmitigated by possible decoding limitations.

Component Skills

Underlying the attainment of proficiency in the various reading outcome skill areas are component skill assets: basic competencies that are necessary to the appearance of reading outcome achievements. These crucial component competencies emerge during early reading development; in order to grow as readers and spellers, children must be able to abstract pertinent sound units in the speech stream, to process print automatically, and to utilize print patterns in order to achieve fluency. Evident in the interface between component and outcome skills is the Matthew effect: Children with the strongest component skill assets tend to display stronger outcome skills, and children who get off to a slow start in reading because of compromised component skills are often caught in a downward spiral of academic failure. Prominent among component skills is *phonological processing* ability, which is crucial to reading success and a concomitant, when impaired, to reading failure. Other key component skills are *automaticity* and *orthographic processing*.

A phonological processing deficit, as we have observed, has been identified as the core deficit in dyslexia. Phonology is the sound system of spoken language; phonological processing involves the abstraction of useful structural units in that system. Phonological awareness is a general awareness of linguistic sound segments; awareness of larger segments such as syllables typically precedes awareness of minimal sound segments or phonemes. The phoneme is the minimal contrastive unit in the sound system of language: the smallest unit that, when replaced, can change meaning. The word *cat*, for instance, is represented phonologically as a sequence of three phonemes. Replacement of any one of those three phonemes affects meaning; thus the words *bat*, *cot*, and *cab* are associated with new meanings.

When children are becoming literate in an alphabetic orthographic system like English, in which phonemes are represented by graphemes—letters or letter clusters—under the alphabetic principle, analysis of the stream of spoken language at a phonemic level is a prerequisite to written-language achievements. Early phonemic awareness permits children to grasp the alphabetic principle; application of that principle in reading and spelling tasks, moreover, calls on phonics knowledge—knowledge of associations between phonemes and graphemes. An understanding of the alphabetic principle and the acquisition of phonics knowledge to apply that principle therefore depend on awareness of phonemes. In order for children to segment the speech stream into its phonemic units and to profit from phonics instruction for reading and spelling, implicit knowledge about the sound structure of spoken language must become explicit. Without direct instructional support, however, explicit awareness of phonemes eludes many young learners. We have seen that the interactions between phonemic awareness and early reading development are bidirectional: Identification of challenge in the component skill area of phonological processing and appropriate instructional intervention will support success in word attack and spelling outcomes, and progress in those areas in turn contributes to further phonemic awareness growth. Without appropriate instruction in phonemic analysis, on the other hand, a prospective reader is vulnerable to the Matthew effect.

The phonological processing abilities of an emerging reader are first manifested in sensitivity at the syllabic and subsyllabic levels: To assess early phonological processing skill, an evaluator might ask a child to tap out syllables in a word, to judge or produce rhymes, or to compare initial or final consonant sounds in words. As reading skills develop, sensitivity at the phonemic level is critical; a child might be asked to segment a syllable into phonemic units, to blend phonemic segments into words, or to manipulate phonemic segments in a syllable (e.g., to say *bed* without /b/). Important, too, in investigations of phonological processing skill level are tests of working phonological memory; a child might be asked to repeat word lists to a supraspan level (a level at which the list length exceeds working-memory span).

As a second component skill, *automaticity* is crucial to growth in written-language outcomes. Automaticity in any process means that the process is rapid, obligatory, and autonomous. Effortlessness and efficiency in any part of a task will constrain the degree to which finite cognitive and attentional resources are depleted; this consequence of automaticity is particularly important in the multilevel reading task. The attentional demands of comprehension increase as the reader matures; it is crucial that the concomitant demands of decoding decrease for the advancing reader. Automaticity has a special status in the double-deficit hypothesis discussed in Chapter 1; Wolf et al. propose that automaticity challenge—a naming-speed deficit—represents a second core deficit in dyslexia, observing that phonological awareness and rapid automatized naming speed each add unique variance in challenged reading performance. On the other hand, Seidenberg advocates a "phonological umbrella" analysis: The core phonological processing deficit observed in dyslexia affects automaticity and/or accuracy (176–177). Supporting the view that the effects of a phonological processing deficit subsume reduced automaticity is the persistent finding of a core phonological processing deficit across dyslexia research; strengthening the separable-deficit approach are research findings, for instance, that the component areas of phonological processing and naming speed are associated differentially with outcome performances in word attack and word identification, with phonological processing behaviors contributing greater variance in word attack outcomes and naming-speed performance the greater factor in word identification outcomes (Wolf et al. 63). Phonological processing capacity would be more critical to decoding accuracy, whereas automaticity would affect reading fluency more directly.

Models diverge, yet the contribution of automaticity to the skilled reading outcome is clear, and the significance of automaticity increases as the maturing reader encounters increasing complexity in textual content. Proficiency in the component skill of automaticity finds its outcome skill reflex in reading fluency: smooth and lucid decoding as the reader addresses connected text. Automaticity is measured in rapid automatized serial naming: Children are asked to name items in a symbol series in which the stimuli might be letters, numbers, colors, or object images. By the end of the first grade, most children are observed to name serialized alphanumeric (number or letter) symbols with greatest automaticity; for children challenged in automaticity, alphanumeric symbol naming is slower, and letter-naming speed shows the greatest lag.

A third component skill area is that of *orthographic processing*. As we saw earlier, research on the neurology of reading points to the roles, independent and interconnected, of phonological processing and orthographic processing in skilled reading. Dehaene refers to the lexical and the phonological reading routes; the systematic selection of the appropriate route characterizes mature and effective reading. The sophisticated reader processes familiar or irregular words as lexical units, moving directly from the orthographic forms to lexically coded meaning and to pronunciation. That skilled reader, however, processes regular and/or unfamiliar print strings phonologically, moving from the orthographic data of letters and letter clusters to associated sounds and then to meaning and pronunciation and thus drawing on associations between phonological and orthographic segments in a step that is bypassed when the lexical route is selected. The cortical site for phonology–orthography integration is the brain's letterbox or visual word form area (Dehaene 65); at this neurological hub, graphemic strings that arrive as input are recoded for orthographic pattern and are then sent on for phonological and semantic interpretation.

As we saw in Chapter 1, the brain site that will become the visual word form area has not yet taken on its specialized letterbox functions in the prereader; it is through the reader's experience with print and reading growth that the area takes on its distinctive and critical role in the integration of orthographic and phonological stimuli (Adams 18). With respect to the development trajectory of the component skill of orthographic processing, it is of interest that, as Adams notes, the area begins to display specialized activity when the emerging reader achieves letter recognition (17). The component skill area of orthographic processing begins to develop in the emerging reader as alphabet letter recognition; Badian demonstrates that letter knowledge is a strong early predictor of later reading achievement (cf. Chall). Adams stresses the significance, over the course of development, of the print word—of Ehri's "sight word," the unitized string for which grapheme–phoneme connections have bonded word spellings to pronunciations and meanings in lexical memory (Ehri 170): "Each time the word is seen, this link will automatically be recalled" (Adams 17). As orthographic sequences recur across these familiar words, orthographic knowledge grows to include the common spelling patterns. Examples of orthographic regularities in English include patterned syllable spellings, such as that of the word-final *consonant-le* syllable in *table* and *little*, or the English orthographic constraint against word-final *v* and *j*. Reading experience and repeated experiences with orthographic sequences promote the development of orthographic processing competency that includes both automatic recognition of a growing set of sight words and a growing awareness of subword orthographic regularities as this third component skill area matures.

The Evaluation of Reading Skills

An assessment design that incorporates evaluation of the component capacities that underlie reading behaviors, of the measurable outcomes that reflect response to instruction, and of the interaction of these component skills and outcome skills is motivated both by developmental considerations and by concerns regarding the Matthew effect. Those readers whose early learning is supported by strong component abilities tend to display stronger outcome skills, whereas readers whose access to literacy is inhibited by challenge in component areas move toward a downward spiral of failure in outcome areas; the gap between their reading achievement and that of peers with component strengths and consequent outcome skill growth will widen over time. That widening disparity among readers' learning trajectories is of great importance; of equal interest, in the evaluation of reading skills, are dissociations within the individual reading profile itself. When assessing, we subscribe to the *concept of individual differences*: the idea that individuals differ along identifiable and measurable dimensions. Assessment of differences extends to measurements within the individual profile.

Diverse assessment instruments permit us to examine the balance of skills that the individual brings to reading instruction—component skills, or *aptitude*—and skills that the individual acquires through instruction—outcome skills, or *achievement*. We use both aptitude and achievement tests to gather information about an individual's status with respect to reading and can then construct an individual reading profile. Aptitude tests measure ability to learn, given the opportunity to do so; they permit us to project future performance as we assess learning capacity and the potential effect of learning experiences. Achievement tests measure what has been learned; they offer a window into present performance as we assess developed capacity: the actual effect of learning experience. As we investigate an individual reading profile, there are appropriate roles, too, for both norm-referenced and criterion-referenced measures: The norm-referenced measure allows us to compare an individual's status to that of other individuals, whereas a criterion-referenced measure allows us to view an individual's position with reference to minimum standards or preestablished criteria in a learning area such as reading.

In addition, we can use both standardized and informal instruments. When we use a standardized test, uniform and controlled testing conditions for administration, materials, and scoring permit test results to yield a valid comparison across individuals: A person responding in the same way as does another person receives the same test score. A standardized, norm-referenced test yields an individual raw score that conveys little information on its own but can be usefully interpreted in a meaningful frame of reference. Interpretation yields an array of derived scores, such as percentile, standard score, grade equivalent, and age equivalent. These derived scores permit us to compare the individual performance to average norming-sample levels. The *percentile* represents the proportion of individuals in the standardization sample whose scores were below a particular test score; the higher the percentile is, the more elevated that person's score is, relative to the scores of (age or grade) peers in the standardization sample. The *standard score* captures the distance from the (age or grade) norming group's mean. The *grade equivalent* matches the individual's performance to the average performance on this test of a group of other students at a particular grade level; the *age equivalent* matches the individual's performance to the average performance, on this test, of a group of other students at a particular age level. A well-designed informal test differs in its flexibility: Testing choices can be guided by testing goals, by student needs, or by individualized assessment questions. The assessor who is administering an informal assessment measure can choose not only to measure performance levels but also to explore process and style; an informal reading inventory can illuminate reading strategy, for instance, as a reader engages with text.

Access to a variety of assessing measures allows us to break down the reading process into narrow skills; no single skill will tell us how a child reads, but we can gain insight into an individual reader's status by understanding reading behavior in terms of an individual profile that is a composite of strengths and challenges, and of parities and discrepancies. After administering a test, scoring test results, and interpreting formal test results as derived scores, the tester can evaluate each formal derived score and informal observation in the context of the full result set, synthesizing parity and discrepancy findings to abstract a reading profile. Of interest are the comparisons between the individual's performance and the performances of others in a standardization sample; of equal importance are the performance-level equivalences and contrasts within the individual reader profile.

The Assessment

Reading evaluation—and an assessment for dyslexia—may be planned for various diagnostic, prognostic, and prescriptive purposes. A clinician, an educator, and/or a caregiver may be seeking to understand an individual's written-language profile and literacy behaviors in order to plan instruction, design treatment, monitor academic progress, or assess the appropriateness of a program; when evaluating for any of these reasons, the evaluator is cognizant of certain premises. There is an inevitable interaction between the individual and the assessment environment; when testing, the evaluator will benefit from a record of observations made during the course of the evaluation. In addition, the evaluator benefits from triangulation of data, such that multiple information sources are consulted. With respect to the objective/quantitative component, the evaluator is subscribing to the concept of individual differences: the assumption that individuals differ along identifiable and measurable dimensions.

In a reading evaluation, those quantifiable dimensions are realized as the narrow skills into which we can break down the reading process; no single skill tells us how an individual reads, but we can understand the complex of literacy behavior outcomes as an individual profile of quantifiable assets and challenges. Measurements may indicate *relative strengths and challenges*: Levels may be greater or lower than others in the individual profile. Measurements may also reflect *absolute strengths and challenges*: They may be elevated or reduced in comparison to the average performance of age or grade peers who were tested on the same set of items under commensurate testing conditions. Test administration, result scoring, score interpretation, and the evaluation of quantitative results and qualitative findings yield a profile comprising performance levels on the various dimensions.

The testing battery that follows reflects the preceding assumptions; its construction is also founded on the premise that both component-skill levels and outcome-skill levels represent key measurements. Component-skill levels predict the efficacy of instruction, and they are explanatory with respect to performance on outcome measures, which in turn indicate the benefit a student has derived from classroom instruction. The testing battery presented here, designed for readers who have begun literacy instruction, translates into roughly two hours of testing and draws on diverse assessment instruments: both formal and informal assessments, and both norm-referenced and criterion-referenced measures. Component skills are assessed on the *Comprehensive Test of Phonological Processing*, second edition, or *CTOPP-2* (Wagner et al.); phonological processing skills and automaticity assets are measured. Outcome skills in single-word decoding are measured on the *Woodcock Reading Mastery Tests*, third edition, or *WRMT-III* (Woodcock); outcome skills in single-word encoding are measured on the *Test of Written Spelling*, fifth edition, or *TWS-5* (Larsen et al.). To assess oral reading fluency and text comprehension, an informal reading inventory, the *Qualitative Reading Inventory*, sixth edition, or *QRI-6* (Leslie and Caldwell) is utilized.

The assessment instruments listed here are used selectively; subtest selections are specified as each instrument is discussed. The battery is designed to diagnose dyslexia, reading challenge that is characterized by reduced component-skill assets in phonological awareness and automaticity and reduced outcome achievements in reading and spelling. The assessment measures address elements that, aggregated, identify dyslexia's specific challenge. The source of this specific challenge—a core deficit in phonological processing—is specific as well, and its immediate impact is circumscribed; thus linguistic comprehension—the second factor, under the simple view of reading, in reading competence—need not be affected. For this reason, it is important to include a linguistic comprehension measure in the battery, in order to distinguish decoding and comprehension as possible sources of reduced reading competence. The two-hour battery can, when appropriate, be administered in a single session; alternatively, the tests can be divided into two (or more) administration groupings. In a first session, for instance, the tester might administer the selections from the *WRMT-III* and the *QRI-6*; in a second session, the *CTOPP-2* selections and the *TWS-5* might be administered. Details on these instruments and on recommended sections and procedures follow.

The *Comprehensive Test of Phonological Processing*

The *Comprehensive Test of Phonological Processing*, second edition (*CTOPP-2*) is an individually administered battery of subtests designed for formal assessment of awareness of, access to, and ability to manipulate phonological structures: spoken-language sound forms. The individual's scores on discrete subtests can be interpreted by comparing raw scores to testing norms; in addition, composite scores in the phonological awareness, phonological memory, and rapid naming areas can be derived. Because the *CTOPP-2* offers two versions, one developed for children between the ages of four and six and the other for individuals between seven and twenty-four years, test results can play diverse roles. As a measure of component skill levels—of aptitudes in areas critical to literacy achievements—the *CTOPP-2* can be administered to individuals who have received reading instruction, in order to assess the degree of neurological preparedness they are bringing to the instructional context. In addition, because the *CTOPP-2* includes norms for very young children who have not yet begun reading instruction, the subtests designed for younger children can be used in screening: Challenged performance in the component skill areas measured on the *CTOPP-2* suggests risk for learning challenge when instruction in reading commences. The *CTOPP-2* subtests that are included in the assessment battery developed here are the *CTOPP-2 core subtests*: Elision, Blending Words, Phoneme Isolation, Memory for Digits, Nonword Repetition, Rapid Digit Naming, and Rapid Letter Naming. Raw scores from these core subtests are utilized to derive scaled scores for the subtests; those subtest scaled scores are used to derive the Phonological Awareness, Phonological Memory, and Rapid Symbolic Naming composite scores.

Phonological Awareness composite score levels reflect capacity to access discrete components of the sound structure of language: to conceptualize and identify the syllabic and phonemic units in spoken words. Adequate phonemic awareness is not only facilitative but also necessary to a mastery of the alphabetic reading and writing code of English and to the achievement of productive word attack, word identification, and spelling skills. Scaled scores derived from the Elision, Blending Words, and Phoneme Isolation subtest raw scores contribute to the Phonological Awareness composite derived scores. In the Elision subtest, the student is asked to indicate the phonological form that remains after designated sounds are omitted from orally presented words; in the Blending Words subtest, the student is asked to form a word from a sequence of individually presented sounds; in Phoneme Isolation, the student is asked to identify a specified sound (the first, last, middle, second, third, or fourth sound) in orally presented words.

Phonological Memory composite score levels reflect the ability to code and store speech input temporarily in working memory, so that language information can be retrieved for and applied to reading and spelling tasks; phonological memory supports the acquisition of new oral and written vocabulary and is drawn on when new words are segmented phonemically for encoding or when their phonemic segments are blended for decoding. Scaled scores derived from the Memory for Digits and Nonword Repetition subtest raw scores are used to calculate the Phonological Memory composite derived scores. In the Memory for Digits subtest, the student is asked to repeat a series of two to eight digit names presented orally at a rate of two digit names per second; in the Nonword Repetition subtest, the student is asked to repeat orally presented nonwords—invented words that are possible but lexically nonexistent English phonological strings—between three and fifteen phonemes in length.

Rapid Symbolic Naming composite score levels reflect automaticity in retrieval of phonological forms associated with graphic symbol stimuli. Rapid retrieval of symbol names has been cited as an important contributor to reading achievement; fluent serial naming competence has been shown to be a strong predictor of reading competence. The role of automaticity as a component skill in the achievement of reading outcome skills was observed earlier; Maryanne Wolf, whose research was instrumental in foregrounding the role of automaticity in both dyslexia and reading skill, has argued (cf. Wolf et al.) that phonological processing and naming speed represent distinctive skill and potential deficit areas for readers, whereas Seidenberg and Shaywitz, for instance, perceive phonological processing as the singular core challenge in dyslexia and position speed and accuracy—automaticity and phonological awareness—under the same "phonological umbrella" (Seidenberg 176). In the *CTOPP-2*, Wagner et al. adopt the latter approach and offer rapid naming assessment to measure performance in one of their three phonological processing skill areas.

Under either model, however, the insight (cf. Wolf et al.) that a naming-speed deficit interacts significantly with reading outcomes has been of profound importance not only in dyslexia research but also in clinical programming, and the *CTOPP-2* Rapid Symbolic Naming composite level is a critical component-skill measure on the assessment battery developed here. Scaled scores based on the Rapid Digit Naming and Rapid Letter Naming subtest raw scores are used to derive the Rapid Symbolic Naming composite derived scores. Those subtests measure the speed and efficiency of processes under which letters and numbers in randomly arranged series are named. In Rapid Digit Naming, the speed with which a student can name numbers in a sequence is measured; in Rapid Letter Naming, the speed with which a student can name letters in a sequence is assessed.

The *CTOPP-2* core subtests permit us to assess component-skill acquisitions, as crucial aspects of a reader's asset/challenge profile. Component-skill levels will predict efficacy of classroom instruction and will indicate current or potential underlying issues; after component-skill assets are investigated, outcome achievements are examined.

The *Woodcock Reading Mastery Tests*

The *Woodcock Reading Mastery Tests*, third edition (*WRMT-III*) represents an individually administered battery of subtests measuring aspects of reading readiness and reading. *WRMT-III* grade-referenced norms are provided for levels from prekindergarten through the twelfth grade; age norms extend from four years, six months, through seventy-nine years, eleven months. Among the nine subtests that make up this formal test battery, the two subtests in the Basic Skills Cluster represent two single-word reading measures: Word Identification and Word Attack. Because these two Basic Skills Cluster subtests measure outcome achievements resulting from academic instruction, age norms begin at six years and grade norms begin at grade one.

The two Basic Skills *WRMT-III* subtests measure reading behaviors associated with two of Ehri's reading development phases: the full alphabetic phase and the consolidated alphabetic phase. When children form "complete connections between letters in spellings and phonemes in pronunciations" (Ehri 174) and word spellings instantiate the knowledge of sound–symbol associations—the phonics knowledge—that they have acquired, developing readers are in the full alphabetic phase and apply their graphophonemic knowledge to decode unfamiliar single words. The Word Attack subtest measures this application skill: The student applies phonics knowledge to read a list of nonwords—invented words that are lexically nonexistent but phonetically and orthographically possible and orthographically transparent, insofar as the systematic application of conventional phonics rules yields a complete and unique pronunciation for the nonword. The Word Identification subtest, in contrast, measures the reading of single, decontextualized real words, a skill associated with Ehri's consolidated alphabetic phase. At this point, a familiar word's orthography is bonded to the word's pronunciation; the orthography is retained in lexical memory and retrieved automatically as a single word unit. Successful and productive single-word reading requires skills both in word attack and in word identification—the fluent retrieval and application of graphophonemic, orthographic, and lexical knowledge—for the decoding of unfamiliar words and the automatic identification of familiar words. Both word-specific lexical knowledge and knowledge of graphophonemic and orthographic regularities are critical, too, to another single-word outcome achievement: spelling.

The *Test of Written Spelling*

The *Test of Written Spelling*, fifth edition (*TWS-5*) is a formal test of spelling achievement that is individually administered in a dictated word format. *TWS-5* grade-referenced norms are provided for the first grade through the twelfth grade; age-referenced norms are provided for six through eighteen years. Spelling and reading outcome skills generally are highly correlated and often progress together in an individual; adequate component skill development in phonemic awareness and a secure base in phonics knowledge are crucial to success in both outcome skill areas.

Like reading skill, spelling skill can be observed to progress through a series of stages. Moats describes the maturation of spelling skills: At four years, the young writer, like the prereader, is unaware of the alphabetic principle and creates ad hoc *precommunicative* print or pseudoprint strings (35). At five years, a *semiphonetic* stance emerges as the writer begins to recognize letters, begins to understand that letters are associated with sounds, and uses letters to represent words, syllables, and sounds (35–36). At five to six years, the child arrives at the *phonetic* stage, acquiring letter names and some sound–symbol associative knowledge. At this stage, the alphabetic insight—the insight that English spelling is founded on the alphabetic principle—appears, and the child represents all speech sounds systematically, with one letter standing for each sound. Spellings are based on sound—on surface phonetic (rather than morphophonemic) features of spoken language—and children can read back their own spellings (37–38). At this point, children benefit from classroom endorsement of their own invented spellings; as children activate their phonemic awareness and phonics knowledge, they internalize the connections between spoken and written language.

It is during the *transitional* stage that follows, at six to seven years, that children's understanding of the connections between speech and print becomes more complicated: Formal spelling instruction introduces young spellers to the overlay of English orthographic conventions interrupting the one-to-one sound–symbol correspondence that would characterize a phonetically transparent orthography. Aware of orthographic features such as silent or doubled letters, and therefore abandoning a simple phonetic approach, the transitional speller produces misspellings that deviate from conventional orthography in unsystematic ways; the transitional speller may appear to be regressing but is in fact moving toward a deeper insight regarding the multiple layers of English orthography. Moats notes that transitional spelling represents "a more advanced approximation of the word ... because it reflects partial orthographic memory" (40). During the *morphophonemic* stage, at seven to eight years, the speller observes that not only phonemes but also morphemes—meaning units—are represented in spellings; the earlier phonetic stance is also enriched by orthographic insights, as the speller appreciates the complex orthographic patterning that is reflected in English print (40).

Maturing, the writer learns that although spelling does not make the demands on lexical retrieval that reading does, it requires accurate grapheme retrieval; phonological and morphological awareness, orthographic knowledge, and phonics knowledge are more heavily relied on in successful spelling. The translation of sound into print in the spelling process, moreover, is less predictable than is the translation of print into sound during reading. Whereas decoding has a singular real-word target, encoding may not: The complex orthography of English may suggest multiple phonetically legitimate letter strings for the encoding of a word, yet only one string will be the conventional choice. Precise word-specific knowledge is therefore required for spelling success. And although spelling is guided by phonetic sequence, we have seen that coarticulation, which permits us to speak and hear as rapidly as we think and thus makes communication possible, camouflages phonemes in a word. For the dyslexic reader/writer, spelling may be more difficult than reading and may be the last challenge to be remediated (Shaywitz 114). Measurement of the single-word outcome skills of word identification, word attack, and spelling is crucial in the construction of the individual reading profile; crucial, too, is assessment of the learner's response to connected text.

The *Qualitative Reading Inventory*

The *Qualitative Reading Inventory*, sixth edition (QRI-6) is an individually administered informal reading inventory that permits the observation of reading behaviors in naturalistic print contexts; it can be used to identify text levels at which successful reading occurs. Supplying materials at the preprimer through the high school reading level, the QRI-6 provides graded word lists, graded passages, and comprehension probes for each passage; these materials can be utilized to assess accuracy and rate in the oral reading of connected text, silent reading skills, reading comprehension, and listening comprehension. At the early levels, the QRI-6 supplies passages with and without illustrations; both narrative and expository reading selections are provided at all levels. The authenticity of the text materials is important; the selections resemble those encountered by students in classroom instruction.

The informal character of the QRI-6 permits the evaluator to select from an array of assessment strategies in order to gain a deep understanding of a reader's response to text, while addressing individualized assessment concerns. To explore the role of content familiarity in a student's text comprehension, the familiarity/unfamiliarity of a selection's content can be evaluated before the selection itself is read; in addition, this informal assessment inventory provides opportunities for the examiner to investigate a student's reading strategies by selecting from a menu of techniques. The examiner may elect to offer the student a *look-back* option during comprehension assessment, for instance, or may explore the student's text apprehension through the *think-aloud* option. The student's oral reading rate can be calculated and then considered in light of expected rate ranges at the various passage levels. And text comprehension can be observed through a *retelling* task, as well as through explicit and implicit comprehension probes.

Because various passage selections are available at each level, the evaluator may also assess both reading comprehension and listening comprehension at a given text level; this opportunity is particular valuable when it is important to distinguish linguistic comprehension from reading comprehension, which may be vitiated by decoding challenge. In the terms of the simple view of reading, under which reading competence is the product of decoding competence and linguistic comprehension competence, reading competence may be compromised by reduced decoding capacity, even in the presence of strong language comprehension skills. In order to avoid an assessment confound, it is crucial that decoding and comprehension measures be dissociated in the assessment context. This dissociation can be achieved through the assessment of listening comprehension: by observing the comprehension of text that has been read aloud to the student.

The informal character of the *QRI-6* makes it a flexible instrument: The examiner can utilize the graded passages in ways that will illuminate a student's reading process and elucidate comprehension assets and challenges. In addition, the *QRI-6* is a criterion-referenced measure. Whereas a norm-referenced test like the *CTOPP-2*, the *WRMT-III*, or the *TWS-5* offers a comparison between an individual's performance and the average performance of an age or grade peer group on the range of test items, a criterion-referenced test allows the evaluator to determine whether an individual's skill level meets criterial standards when performance is measured on graded material. In the case of the *QRI-6*, the criterion-referenced assessment permits measurement of a student's reading performance against texts whose difficulty level conforms to graded academic expectations; the text level at which the student will read and comprehend successfully in a learning context can be identified.

Three performance levels can be derived on the *QRI-6*: the *independent*, *instructional*, and *frustration* levels. If a student reads a new passage with 90–97 percent accuracy, the student is *instructional*, from a decoding perspective, at that passage level: For decoding purposes, a similarly leveled passage would be an appropriate selection for that reader's classroom instruction. If a student reads a new passage with 98 percent (or greater) accuracy, the student is *independent*, from a decoding perspective, at that passage level: A similarly leveled passage would be an apt choice, from a decoding perspective, for independent reading. Decoding accuracy below 90 percent will position the reader at *frustration* level; the passage is too advanced, from a decoding angle, for that student's classroom instruction.

In order for a passage to be fully appropriate for a reader, however, comprehension must be considered. The *QRI-6* provides passage comprehension questions that allow the examiner to determine whether comprehension of an administered passage is at an independent level (questions are answered with 90 percent or greater success), at an instructional level (questions are answered with 67–89 percent success), or at a frustration level (questions are answered with less than 67 percent success). The examiner can then determine whether a student's overall reading competence on a given passage is in the independent, instructional, or frustration range, utilizing both the decoding performance and the comprehension performance to calculate the total passage reading performance. Performance measures on the graded passage on which the reader has been identified as instructional for overall reading include the rate (words per minute) measure; the student's performance figure can be compared to typical-range figures for each grade, provided in the *QRI-6* manual.

In the context of an assessment of a student's assets, challenges, and component and outcome skill acquisitions, the examiner can utilize the *QRI-6* to determine the text level at which the student's overall reading competence is instructional and then the text level at which the student's listening comprehension is instructional. When a dyslexia diagnosis is under consideration, assessment of comprehension in the listening modality is crucial to a disengagement of decoding and linguistic comprehension; listening comprehension measurement allows the examiner to rule out the possible impact of decoding challenge on the student's language comprehension performance. To determine the student's comprehension level when decoding demands are removed, the examiner administers comprehension questions on a passage that the student has listened to. On that graded passage on which the student has been identified as instructional for listening comprehension, the examiner may administer a retelling measure; the resulting passage recall level may be viewed in light of the (provided) typical range for the passage level. Measurement of listening comprehension will help the examiner to develop a coherent written-language profile, assembling results derived on diverse instruments in order to aggregate the component-skill and outcome-skill performance levels that represent the student's response to written text.

The Written-Language Evaluation

The written-language evaluation battery described here has a theoretical base in research on reading development and on its disruption. We observed that the first challenge for a new reader is one that all readers face: Mastery of the literacy skills of reading and writing requires that implicit knowledge of spoken language be made explicit. Children are prepared neurologically to acquire the natural system of spoken language, but literacy is achieved through direct instruction, and literacy growth is conditional: Mastery of the alphabetic orthographic code of English requires that the learner be able to segment the speech stream phonemically. This phonemic segmentation requirement complicates the early entry into literacy, and that complication is significant for the dyslexic learner: Dyslexia's core phonological processing deficit makes phonemic segmentation particularly challenging.

That special challenge underscores the vital role of early assessment, identification, and treatment for the dyslexic student. The assessment battery described here is grounded in the model of the simple view of reading, under which reading competence is the product of decoding competence and comprehension competence. The assessment battery includes outcome measures of decoding and of linguistic comprehension; it also includes a spelling measure, insofar as encoding presents a special challenge for the dyslexic learner. In addition, component measures permit an assessment of the underlying phonological processing and automaticity skills that are necessary to successful achievement of literacy outcomes. Outcome-skill assessment provides a window into the results of instruction; component-skill assessment illuminates the capacities that the learner brings to the instructional context. Together, measures of component capacities and outcome achievements illuminate contours of the individual written-language profile.

Works Cited

Adams, Marilyn Jager. "The Relation Between Alphabetic Basics, Word Recognition, and Reading." *What Research Has to Say About Reading Instruction.* Eds. S. Jay Samuels and Alan E. Farstrup. Newark, DE: International Reading Association, 2011. 4–24.

Badian, Nathlie. "Predicting Reading Ability over the Long Term: The Changing Roles of Letter Naming, Phonological Awareness, and Orthographic Processing." *Annals of Dyslexia* 45 (1995): 79–96.

Cassar, Marie, Rebecca Treiman, Louisa Moats, Tatiana Cury Pollo, and Brett Kessler. "How Do the Spellings of Children with Dyslexia Compare with Those of Nondyslexic Children?" *Reading and Writing* 18 (2005): 27–49.

Chall, Jeanne. *Stages of Reading Development.* New York: McGraw-Hill, 1983.

Dehaene, Stanislas. *Reading in the Brain.* New York: Penguin, 2009.

Ehri, Linnea. "Learning to Read Words." *Scientific Studies of Reading* 9:2 (2005): 167–188.

Gough, Philip B., and William E. Tunmer. "Decoding, Reading, and Reading Disability." *Remedial and Special Education* 7:1 (1986): 6–10.

Hoover, Wesley A., and Philip B. Gough. "The Simple View of Reading." *Reading and Writing: An Interdisciplinary Journal* 2 (1990): 127–160.

Kennedy, Becky. "Hyperlexia Profiles." *Brain and Language* 84 (2003): 204–221.

Larsen, Stephen C., Donald D. Hammill, and Louisa C. Moats. *TWS-5: Test of Written Spelling* (5th ed.). Austin, TX: Pro-Ed, 2013.

Leslie, Lauren, and JoAnne Caldwell. *QRI-6: Qualitative Reading Inventory* (6th ed.). Boston, MA: Pearson, 2017.

Moats, Louisa Cooke. *Spelling: Development, Disability, and Instruction.* Timonium, MD: York Press, 1995.

Seidenberg, Mark. *Language at the Speed of Sight.* New York: Basic Books, 2017.

Shaywitz, Sally. *Overcoming Dyslexia.* New York: Vintage Books, 2005.

Stanovich, Keith. "Matthew Effects in Reading: Some Consequences of Individual Differences in the Acquisition of Literacy." *Reading Research Quarterly* 21:4 (Fall 1986): 360–407.

Treffert, Darold A. "Hyperlexia III: Separating 'Autistic-like' Behaviors from Autistic Disorder: Assessing Children Who Read Early or Speak Late." *Wisconsin Medical Journal* 110:6 (2011): 281–286.

Tunmer, William, and Keith Greaney. "Defining Dyslexia." *Journal of Learning Disabilities* 43:3 (2010): 229–243.

Wagner, Richard K., Joseph K. Torgesen, Carol A. Rashotte, and Nils A. Pearson. *CTOPP-2: Comprehensive Test of Phonological Processing* (2nd ed.). Austin, TX: Pro-Ed, 2013.

Wolf, Maryanne, Alyssa Goldberg O'Rourke, Calvin Gidney, Maureen Lovett, Paul Cirino, and Robin Morris. "The Second Deficit: An Investigation of the Independence of Phonological and Naming-Speed Deficits in Developmental Dyslexia." *Reading and Writing: An Interdisciplinary Journal* 15 (2002): 43–72.

Woodcock, Richard W. *WRMT-III: Woodcock Reading Mastery Tests* (3rd ed.). San Antonio, TX: Pearson, 2011.

3 The Written-Language Profile

Dyslexia and the Individual

An inspection of dyslexia's clinical presentation and the exploration of linguistic and neurological contingencies underlying written-language challenge point to generalizations about dyslexia. Research findings converge on the localization of dyslexia's source: A core deficit in phonological processing—in the processing of spoken language's minimal sound segment—that does not affect the acquisition of spoken language will compromise the learner's entry into literacy. Reading instruction in which the learner is presented with a set of conventional associations between minimal speech units—*phonemes*—and minimal print units—individual letters or letter clusters, or *graphemes*—is ineffective if the phoneme itself is inaccessible: if the learner cannot abstract the phoneme in the context of the speech stream and thus cannot access the phonemic level of language structure. That phonological processing challenge, which does not affect performance in those speaking and listening classroom activities that do not reference print, renders basic reading and spelling performances arduous or impossible. And the pattern of academic challenges accompanying dyslexia has its correlate in a pattern of neurological activity associated with print processing that displays a distinctive developmental trajectory. Dyslexia's "neural signature" (Shaywitz 82) features reduced activation in cortical areas at the back of the brain that typically process phonology and orthography for reading, whereas a characteristic compensating overactivation increases over time in frontal cortical areas that handle reading inefficiently.

These features of dyslexia—of its etiology and its characteristic outcomes—accompany consequences stemming from a core deficit that is specific and is circumscribed. The singular phonological processing deficit, moreover, is situated in an individual bearing a unique array of personal and intellectual assets. In written-language assessment, therefore, we seek to identify the individual profile: to explore the distributional contours of resources and challenges and to observe the transactions among assets and deficits in the dynamic context of the individual. The construct of the individual profile is based on a tenet of reading evaluation: The concept of individual differences offers the insight that individual readers differ along identifiable and measurable skill dimensions; skill levels interact dynamically, moreover, in the reading process. After administering test measures and arriving at a set of results, the evaluator focuses on the interpretation of those results in order to understand the individual dynamic: to learn how the student engages with literacy.

Score Interpretation

Administration of selected measures from the *CTOPP-2*, the *WRMT-III*, the *TWS-5*, and the *QRI-6* permits the evaluator, building on the concept of individual differences, to construct the individual reader's profile of assets and challenges. No single measurement tells us how an individual reads, but the aggregated component- and outcome-skill measurements illuminate the skill complex that represents an individual's literacy function. The skills that make up that composite can be compared to one another and identified as relative assets or challenges when the individual engages with text; measured skills can also be classed as absolute strengths or vulnerabilities according to external valuation. That valuation might utilize norms—average performance levels of (age or grade) peer groups on the same material—or criteria—preestablished standards (e.g., for achievement at grade levels) in a learning area. We have seen that the criterion-referenced *QRI-6* offers the latter interpretive reference: Performance levels are interpreted by measuring them against grade-based standards. Decoding and comprehension performances are interpreted as independent-level, instruction-level, or frustration-level performance on graded text; rate (word–per-minute figures) and recall (percentage of idea units retained from a text) are measured for consistency with graded ranges.

The *CTOPP-2*, the *WRMT-III*, and the *TWS-5*, on the other hand, utilize the first type of interpretive reference. Raw scores achieved through test administration convey little information on their own but are interpreted with reference to test norms; the student's performance is compared to performance in a norming group of peers to whom the test was administered, and the resulting scores are *derived* scores. Those test norms will be age-based norms if the peers are age-mates; they will be grade-based norms if the peers are grade-mates. Certain tests, such as the *WRMT-III*, provide norms by age and by grade; others, such as the *CTOPP-2*, utilize age for norming purposes. It is suggested that age-based norms be used to interpret raw-score results on all three standardized instruments discussed here: the *CTOPP-2*, the *WRMT-III*, and the *TWS-5*. Age-based norms are appropriate when we interpret raw scores on tests of aptitude, such as the *CTOPP-2*, or when we compare aptitude and achievement levels. Because parallels and discrepancies between component-skill (aptitude) levels and outcome-skill (achievement) measurements are of great interest in the assessment of written-language skills, it is suggested that age-based rather than grade-based norms be used to interpret test results when both norm types are (as on the *WRMT-III*) available.

Among derived scores, the percentile represents the ranking approach: Under age-based norms, the percentile score ranks the student relative to age peers. One-half—50 percent—of the group will rank between the 25th and the 75th percentiles, and this range is the average range; a score ranking a student below the 25th percentile places the student below the average range for age, and a score positioning the student above the 75th percentile indicates performance above the average range. The standard score reflects the distance between the student's score and the mean (average) score of age peers. If the mean or average score in the group is 100, one-half of all standard scores will fall between 90 and 110; a standard score below 90 or greater than 110 indicates, respectively, performance below or performance above the average range for age. Age- and grade-equivalent scores represent a matching approach: The age or grade equivalent indicates the norming sample's age or grade level at which the average score in the norming sample matches the score obtained by the student. Age and grade equivalents are often requested on an assessment; crucially, however, they must be clearly explained and understood. An age- or grade-equivalent figure does not signify that a student has criterial skills or content mastery expected at that age or grade level; instead, it signifies that the student's score on the set of test items matched the average score of norming-sample students at that particular age or grade level. Derived scores play a key role in the interpretation of assessment data. Complementing the insights they provide into the individual reader's status with respect to norming-sample performances or criterion-based expectations, moreover, is the information that can be garnered in a close analysis of individual test-item responses.

Response Interpretation

Result figures represent key data in the construction of the student's written-language profile. In addition, the assessment yields rich data in the form of item responses that elucidate both literacy level and strategy. The *QRI-6* incorporates various assessment options in its flexible procedures; the evaluator can make choices that best fit the testing goals, choosing between familiar and unfamiliar passage content, expository or narrative text structure, and passages with or without accompanying images. Another assessment choice is the think-aloud option, under which the evaluator asks the student to pause at designated places while reading a passage and think aloud, articulating responses to the immediate text. This strategy provides the evaluator with a window into the student's processing of textual content.

Comprehension is explored in different ways. After reading or listening to a graded passage, the student may be asked to provide an oral recapitulation of content, as if telling the story to someone who has never heard it. The examiner, interested in the student's capacity to retrieve content elements, is also alert to structure in the student's retelling discourse: Does the student reference story structure when recalling a narrative text? When recalling expository content, does the student distinguish key and supporting ideas? Comprehension questions are then administered in order to probe apprehension of both explicit and implicit textual content. Responses on both the retelling task and the narrative probes offer a window into linguistic comprehension; in an assessment for dyslexia, it is important to evaluate performance in both decoding and language comprehension in order to measure the respective contributions of the two factors to the overall reading outcome. In both the retelling and the comprehension probe tasks, however, memory plays a major role in student performance; the examiner is exploring the student's capacity for and strategy in content retrieval without textual support. To disengage comprehension and memory—to isolate the effects of linguistic comprehension, that is—the evaluator may take advantage of the look-back option, inviting the student to look back at the text in order to answer a comprehension probe. The evaluator thereby shifts the task demand such that apprehension of rather than memory for content is evaluated.

These *QRI-6* choices are built into the informal inventory's format and permit the evaluator to observe, for instance, whether the student is sensitive to content familiarity or text structure, or whether the student is challenged by a confrontational memory demand but draws on a deep understanding of content and profits from the look-back option. In addition, the examiner, attending to the particulars of the student's decoding responses on the *QRI-6*, might consider whether decontextualized single-word decoding (on graded word lists) or decoding in textual context is more successful. The student's responses also offer opportunities for *miscue*—decoding error—analysis; the evaluator is interested in error type. A self-correction when decoding, for instance, is counted as a decoding error on the *QRI-6*, yet self-correction suggests that the reader is self-monitoring, whereas a simple word-omission or substitution error would not.

Unlike the informal *QRI-6*, a formal instrument like the *WRMT-III* or the *TWS-5* is not designed to offer the examiner a chance to make individualized procedural decisions during the assessment process. As on the *QRI-6*, however, decoding and spelling responses to formal test items provide opportunities for error analysis. Learner strategies are reflected in error patterns on the *WRMT-III* Word Identification and Word Attack subtests, as the examiner considers whether the student has achieved automatic sight-word access, for instance, to small common words on the Word Identification subtest, or applies phonics rules systematically and automatically in the Word Attack subtest. In both real-word and nonword decoding, it would be of interest to observe whether the student is seeking a real-word target, for instance, or uses an orthographic chunking strategy, or reveals insecure or partial phonics knowledge.

In the spelling responses on *TWS-5* test items, the examiner might observe whether the student produces a written spelling with automaticity; in addition, the *TWS-5* misspellings might feature errors that are predominantly *dysphonetic* (phonetically implausible) or errors that are *dyseidetic* (conforming to phonological sequence while ignoring distinctive orthographic patterns). A dysphonetic spelling of "mother," for instance, might be *mroth*; a dyseidetic spelling might be *muthr*. And a spelling of that term that showed no sound mediation, with the speller proceeding directly from meaning to print, might be *mom*. In an analysis of spelling responses, sensitivity to the stages of spelling development is meaningful; under Moats's analysis, for instance, the child moves from a phonetic stage through a transitional stage before arriving at the greater sophistication of the morphophonemic spelling stage. Spellings at the transitional stage may appear to ignore sound sequence; rather than indicating an inability to represent phonetic sequences in orthography, however, such spellings may instead signify that the learner has begun to acknowledge the deep character of English orthography. Thus the phonetic speller might spell "walked" as *wokt*, whereas the transitional speller might produce *wlaked*, in a response that appears regressive but foreshadows a more sophisticated awareness of a silent letter in an orthographic pattern. Drawing on the record of student responses to test items, the evaluator can discover patterned literacy behaviors that shed light on an individual's developmental status, strategic approach, and processing style when engaging with print.

The Individual Profile

During the written-language assessment, the student provides a wealth of data when responding to language and to text. The *CTOPP-2* results register crucial component-skill assets and challenges in phonological awareness, phonological memory, and automaticity that the student brings to the instructional context; results on the *WRMT-III*, the *TWS-5*, and the *QRI-6* identify achievements and liabilities in outcome-skill areas, indicating the student's capacity to benefit from instruction. Derived scores and criterial achievement indices allow the evaluator to interpret the results by measuring test performances against developmental expectations and standards. Derived score levels that are above or below the average range indicate strengths and challenges that are absolute: In the academic context, the student who outperforms or is outperformed by average-range (the middle 50 percent of) peers is at an absolute advantage or disadvantage, respectively, in the classroom. This holds for both component-skill (aptitude) and outcome-skill (achievement) measures.

For example, a *TWS-5* standard score (by age) of 85 would reflect an absolute challenge in the outcome area of encoding. The associated percentile level is the 16th percentile; these derived scores indicate that when spelling the set of *TWS-5* test items, the student performed at a level below the average range for norming-population age peers who were tested on the same item set and was outperformed by 84 percent of those age peers. In contrast, other strengths and challenges may be relative. Let us suppose that the fourth-grade student who achieved a standard score of 85 on the *TWS-5* was observed to be instructional at grade level—at level 4—on the *QRI-6*, and that the fourth-grade student was found to be instructional for listening comprehension on level 6 text. The *WRMT-III* Word Attack standard score, on the other hand, was 91, with that performance positioning the student at the 27th percentile for age. This last score falls within the average range: Nonword decoding, as measured on the *WRMT-III* Word Attack subtest, does not represent an absolute challenge. In the context of the *QRI-6* reading outcomes featured in the student's overall written-language profile, however, the Word Attack score reflects a relative challenge for this student and suggests a relative vulnerability—for this student—in nonword decoding. This relative challenge is apparent in light of the student's unexpectedly strong listening comprehension when written text was read aloud. The written-language profile is a composite structure—the composite of component aptitudes and outcome achievements—and that profile features assets and challenges, perhaps absolute and perhaps relative, in the array of literacy behaviors.

To view absolute and relative strengths and challenges in the context of the overall individual profile, consider the representation of this student's profile in his score summary. At nine years, nine months, Hayden was assessed for written-language skills on the test battery described here. The results are summarized in Table 3.1.

Hayden's score set, revealing both absolute and relative assets and challenges in the reading profile, also displays performance contrasts. In an

Table 3.1 Summary of Testing, Grade 4

Name	Age	Grade		
Hayden	9-9	4		
Instrument	**Grade Equivalent**	**Age Equivalent**	**Standard Score**	**Percentile**
CTOPP-2				
Phonological Awareness			88	21
Phonological Memory			88	21
Rapid Symbolic Naming			95	37
WRMT-III				
Word Identification	3.6	9-1	94	34
Word Attack	3.1	8-7	91	27
TWS-5	3.0	8-3	85	16
QRI-6	Overall reading: Instructional on level 4 text			
	Listening comprehension: Instructional on level 6 text			
	Rate on level 4 text: 60 WPM			

individual profile in which certain outcome skills—measured as *WRMT-III* Word Attack performance and *QRI-6* overall reading level—either are in the average range for age or are at an instructional level for the student's assigned grade, other skills are divergent. Thus, for instance, listening comprehension is instructional at two levels above assigned grade: When decoding demands were absent, Hayden's text comprehension advanced substantially beyond grade-level expectations. A score split in which decoding skills and comprehension skills are discrepant is particularly meaningful in reading assessment, especially if academic performance has suggested dyslexia. The overall passage reading level on the *QRI-6* factors in both decoding and reading comprehension skills, but the listening comprehension task offers a more direct measure of the linguistic comprehension factor (C) in reading competence, under the simple view of reading (R = D × C). Recalling Gough and Tunmer's statement that "reading ability should be predictable from a measure of decoding ability (e.g., the ability to pronounce pseudowords) and a measure of *listening* comprehension" (7), we see that the administration of listening comprehension as a separate *QRI-6* task permits the examiner to segregate the measurement of language comprehension in the context of reading assessment.

Following Gough and Tunmer, we can also look more closely at the *WRMT-III* Word Attack subtest performance in this example profile. Although the derived scores associated with that performance position Hayden in the average range for age, the performance measurement falls at the lower end of that average range, suggesting a discrepancy between the two reading factors: Whereas listening comprehension assessment reveals C (language comprehension) to be at a level well above grade expectations, D (decoding) is only narrowly within the average range for age. This contrast suggests, in turn, that D may be limiting R in the *QRI-6* overall reading performance.

In light of Hayden's profile, we might revisit his *TWS-5* result. Because *TWS-5* derived scores positioned Hayden below the average range for age, the spelling outcome measure indicates an absolute challenge. In the context of Hayden's profile, moreover, spelling level contrasts not only with the especially strong *QRI-6* listening comprehension performance but also with the *QRI-6* overall reading performance level. Overall reading performance is instructional on grade-level (level 4) text; on a par with that *QRI-6* result, moreover, is Hayden's *WRMT-III* Word Identification subtest performance. Derived scores on that measure of decontextualized real-word identification are also in the average range for age: The Word Identification standard score is 94, positioning Hayden in the 34th percentile for age. Word identification emphasizes the automatic retrieval of a word's pronunciation in response to the word-specific orthographic pattern; phonemic awareness and secure phonics knowledge support successful word identification (Ehri 174), and alphabet knowledge serves as "a powerful mnemonic" (Ehri 172), yet automatic access to word-specific lexical knowledge drives successful sight-word reading. Less divergent from spelling, however, is nonword decoding level, reflected in the *WRMT-III* Word Attack score. Although the latter performance is also within the average range, it falls at the lower end of that range, suggesting relative vulnerability in the application of phonics knowledge to decode novel and orthographically transparent strings. In nonword reading—as in the decoding of an unfamiliar real word—the reader applies phonics rules automatically to recode print phonologically without the support of stored word knowledge that is invoked in sight-word identification. Successful word attack presupposes full mastery of and automatic access to the set of graphophonemic associations (Ehri 174); it also depends on well-developed phonological processing competence. In order to associate symbols and sounds systematically for word attack, the reader must be able to abstract the phoneme. The same requirement holds for spelling: Phonetic spelling skill requires phoneme awareness and may be even more difficult than reading for the dyslexic student.

We see not only contrasts but also parities in the individual profile; in this sample profile, there is a correspondence between word attack results and those for spelling. As an effect of the core phonological processing deficit in dyslexia (cf., e.g., Adams, Seidenberg, Shaywitz), component skills in phonological processing, foundational to literacy outcome achievements, are vitiated. These skills are measured on the *CTOPP-2*; those performances that most directly reflect phonemic awareness level are included in the Phonological Awareness Composite. That test composite comprises three subtests designed to measure the ability to abstract and manipulate phonemic units: Elision, Blending Words, and Phoneme Isolation. Of these three subtests, the first and the third—Elision and Phoneme Isolation—gauge with particular sensitivity the phonological processing assets required for successful reading and spelling. As noted in the previous chapter, Wolf et al. observed the contribution of phonological processing to variance in word attack outcomes; that correspondence between results on phonological processing measures and results of word attack testing also appears in the assessment context. This clinically observed correspondence extends to spelling measurement: Performances on word attack, spelling, and phonological processing tasks characteristically march together. Of the various phonological processing tasks, Elision and Phoneme Isolation yield results most consistent with those on word attack and spelling measures, with Elision, calling for phonological manipulation, an especially strong predictor of word attack and spelling skill levels.

Hayden's score set, which includes results not only from outcome skill testing but also from component skill assessment, reveals not only the familiar correspondence between spelling and word attack results but also the parity, predicted by research findings and observed clinically, across results on elision, word attack, and spelling tasks. On the *CTOPP-2*, Hayden's standard scores on the Phonological Awareness, Phonological Memory, and Rapid Symbolic Naming Composites are, respectively, 88

(21st percentile for age), 88 (21st percentile), and 95 (25th percentile). *CTOPP-2* subtest derived scores (not displayed in the score set) appear as scaled scores from 1 to 20, centered at 10; within the Phonological Awareness Composite, Hayden's Elision scaled score is 7 (16th percentile), the Phoneme Isolation scaled score is 8 (25th percentile), and the Blending scaled score is 9 (37th percentile). These results, consistent again with expectations founded on research data and clinical patterns, confirm the critical predictive relationship between component skill levels and outcome measurements. A deficit in the component-skill area of phonological processing, reflected most sensitively in performance on the elision task, is associated with outcome reductions in those areas in which performance most directly depends on the phonemic insight: in word attack and spelling.

The contours of Hayden's profile, reflecting assets, challenges, contrasts, and correspondences across testing results, suggest answers to a fundamental assessment question: *How does this student respond to text?* At the same time, new questions are raised. Except for a spelling outcome falling below the average range for age and a listening comprehension outcome at an unexpectedly high level, outcome skill performances are within the average range for age or at criterial level for assigned grade. The contrasts in Hayden's profile, however, are as important as is the appearance of outcome-skill performance results that are consistent, for the most part, with age and grade expectations. Although both single-word reading subtests yielded average-range results, the discrepancy between decoding level and the comprehension level that was displayed when decoding demands were removed is highly suggestive. That discrepancy hints that phonological processing challenge stands between Hayden and the achievement of reading at a level commensurate with language comprehension potential. Hayden's fluency measure when reading level 4 text on the *QRI-6* suggests that oral reading is effortful: The measured reading rate, at 60 words per minute, is within the range expected for students who are instructional on level 4 text—57–115 words per minute—but falls at the lower end of that range. Fluency, like nonword decoding, represents a relative challenge for Hayden.

That phonological processing is not merely a relative area of need but is, in fact, an absolute challenge is apparent when component skill levels are considered: The Phonological Awareness Composite and Phonological Memory Composite performance levels are below the average range for age. Within the Phonological Awareness Composite, absolute challenge was reflected on the Elision subtest result; as we observed, elision has been shown in research and in clinical observation to be a strong predictor of word attack and spelling results. Reduced, too, are scores for the Phonological Memory Composite. Research (cf., e.g., Morais and Mousty) has revealed reciprocity between development in the component-skill area of phonological awareness and outcome-skill growth in reading and spelling: Not only does intervention ameliorating the consequences of a phonological awareness deficit improve reading and spelling outcomes (cf., e.g., Vellutino and Fletcher, Adams), but decoding advances also support phonological awareness growth. The possibility of change in the component skill itself, the distal effect of a change on literacy, and a bidirectional relationship between component-skill advances and outcome-skill growth are not observed, however, in the case of phonological memory. Melby-Lervag et al., in a meta-review of studies of working-memory training programs, conclude that such training programs may induce temporary memory changes but do not show transfer effects in higher-level skill areas like reading. Unlike phonological awareness skills, phonological memory skills do not seem to be remediable, and they do not seem to be impacted by remediation in reading. Literacy growth may support the development of phonological awareness, but reduced phonological memory is more likely to remain at a low level.

Does Hayden's profile suggest dyslexia? We can appose the assessment results and the IDA's definition of dyslexia, repeated here:

> Dyslexia is a specific learning disability that is neurobiological in origin. It is characterized by difficulties with accurate and/or fluent word recognition and by poor spelling and decoding abilities. These difficulties typically result from a deficit in the phonological component of language that is often unexpected in relation to other cognitive abilities and the provision of effective classroom instruction. Secondary consequences may include problems in reading comprehension and reduced reading experience that can impede growth of vocabulary and background knowledge.
>
> (International Dyslexia Association, 2002; see Lyon et al. 2)

The absolute challenge in spelling indicated by Hayden's *TWS-5* results is consistent with the reference to spelling in the IDA definition, as is the absolute challenge in phonological awareness reflected in the *CTOPP-2* assessment. The unexpectedness of these challenges in Hayden's profile is revealed not only in the contrast with reading skills that are in the average range for age and indicate that Hayden is instructional on grade-level text, but also in collocation with the special comprehension strength documented through *QRI-6* listening comprehension assessment. In the context of Hayden's profile, the deficit in phonological processing that is the putative source of the reduced spelling performance is a circumscribed deficit.

Given average-range performance in single-word reading and instructional status on grade-level connected text, however, can an individual be identified as dyslexic? Hayden's academic history would be pertinent here. When Hayden was seven years old and in the second grade, an assessment was also completed. The results of that earlier assessment appear in Table 3.2.

At age seven years, eleven months, Hayden was instructional for overall reading on illustrated primer text—text at the first-grade level—although

Table 3.2 Summary of Testing, Grade 2

Name	Age	Grade		
Hayden	7-11	2		
Instrument	**Grade Equivalent**	**Age Equivalent**	**Standard Score**	**Percentile**
CTOPP-2				
Phonological Awareness			84	14
Phonological Memory			88	21
Rapid Symbolic Naming			98	45
WRMT-III				
Word Identification	1.3	6-8	80	9
Word Attack	1.4	6-10	87	19
TWS-5	<1.0	6-9	85	16
QRI-6	Overall reading: Instructional on primer text			
	Listening comprehension: Instructional on level 3 text			
	Rate on primer text: 19 WPM			

listening comprehension was at an instructional level on level 3 material. When he read primer text orally, his reading rate, at 19 words per minute, was below the expected range for students who are instructional at that level. Single-word reading and spelling performances reflected absolute challenge in those areas. Hayden's standard score by age on the *WRMT-III* Word Identification subtest was 80, placing him in the 9th percentile in his norming age group. His Word Attack subtest standard score was 87 (19th percentile), and spelling on the *TWS-5* earned a standard score (by age) of 85 (16th percentile). On the *CTOPP-2*, Phonological Awareness and Phonological Memory Composite standard scores were 84 (14th percentile) and 88 (21st percentile), respectively; the Rapid Symbolic Naming standard score, at 98 (45th percentile), was the only assessment score that fell within the average or expected range for age.

Hayden's mother and father, a doctor and an engineer, had both faced reading challenges as children; when the evaluator reviewed the testing results with them and diagnosed dyslexia, he suggested that they seek out an Orton–Gillingham reading therapist. The Orton–Gillingham approach is a code-based, sequential, multisensory treatment program; letter sounds and sound–symbol associations are taught explicitly, with persistent training in phoneme segmentation, sound blending, decoding, and encoding. Hayden began to receive an hour of individual reading therapy administered thrice weekly. Hayden's predilection for reading and listening to text represented an advantage: His immersion in literacy activities worked to counter the potential downward spiral of the Matthew effect. The highly structured treatment program proved to be the right choice; two years later, the assessment results indicated substantial growth, with Hayden achieving results in the average range for age on single-word reading tasks and instructional status on grade-level text.

However, the markers of a phonological processing deficit remain apparent in Hayden's profile. The contours of that profile continue to register the effects of that deficit in both component and outcome skill areas: in persistent challenge in phonological awareness, phonological memory, and spelling tasks. The neural source—the "neural signature" (Shaywitz 82) for the core phonological processing challenge that compromises written-language achievement in students like Hayden—is inscribed not only in neural architecture but also in neural circuitry and development. Hayden's case demonstrates, however, that the effects of dyslexia need be neither intractable nor immutable. Our human brain, vulnerable to the contingencies of neurological difference, is also the neural source of ingenious research efforts, profound insights, and clinical acumen; as we advance in our understanding of the cortical mapping of literacy challenge, we grow in our sophistication at retraining and recircuiting print processes (Shaywitz 85–86). Component-skill areas like phonological memory may be obdurate, with respect to remediation; others, however, such as phonemic awareness, can profit from a bidirectional relationship with literacy development. And challenged students who, like Hayden, bring gifts like superior comprehension and a love for text, are positioned to confound and to reverse the Matthew effect, as treatment opens the door for the reading practice that is critical to reading growth.

Diagnosing Dyslexia

Shaywitz characterizes the scientific approach to the evaluation for and diagnosis of dyslexia as "organic" (137): Assessment practice is enriched by the contributions of science, by sensitivity to the personal profile and developmental history, by the consultation of multiple information sources, and by thoughtful attention to the understanding of dyslexia reflected in the IDA's 2002 definition. She highlights necessary features of the assessment: A reduction in reading performance relative to age and to educational experience should be documented, and that reduction should have the unexpected character cited in the IDA statement: Reduced reading skill should represent, in the array of cognitive assets, a challenge that is circumscribed and that persists in spite of effective classroom instruction. In the diagnosis of dyslexia, the evaluator will note a characteristic pattern in written-language outcome skill measurements; Shaywitz cites word identification difficulty, word attack challenge, slow reading rate, and challenged spelling, with reading comprehension at a higher level. The evaluator should document, too, a phonological processing challenge; here, Shaywitz adduces the CTOPP-2 subtests as effective diagnostic measures (132–137).

Hayden's evaluation follows Shaywitz's model. In the first evaluation, completed when Hayden was in the second grade, reading performance that was reduced relative to grade and instructional expectations was documented at the single-word level and on connected text. Reduction was observed in both rate and accuracy; reduced spelling skill was documented as well. The unexpectedness of the reading challenge was apparent in the disparity between Hayden's documented decoding level and an elevated linguistic comprehension capacity, revealed in his *QRI-6* listening comprehension performance; *CTOPP-2* subtest administration showed a phonological processing deficit. The characteristic patterning of testing results pointed to a diagnosis of dyslexia; that diagnosis, guided by evaluation data, was consistent with data from other sources—such as the record of familial history of reading challenge. The events that followed—the individualized clinical response and Hayden's positive response to treatment—revealed the soundness of the diagnosis. The recommendation of Orton–Gillingham treatment was especially appropriate in the context of Hayden's individual profile, featuring special comprehension strength and an affinity for literacy. Two years later, evaluation revealed that reading at the single-word and textual levels was within the average range for age or at the appropriate level for assigned grade, although a discrepancy remained between decoding achievement and elevated linguistic comprehension. Hayden's positive response to intervention tailored to a dyslexia diagnosis confirms the aptness of that diagnosis.

Reference has been made, throughout this discussion of the written-language profile, to the diagnostic significance of both parities and discrepancies within that profile. In the context of an observed decoding performance reduction in an evaluation for dyslexia, the pertinence of a score split between decoding and comprehension skills was underscored, insofar as that split reflected the unexpected character of the decoding challenge. In the discussion of Hayden's written-language profile at nine years, a performance discrepancy between listening comprehension and overall reading was, likewise, noteworthy, because it highlighted the elevation in text comprehension when performance was unconstrained by decoding demands. Historically, a (different) discrepancy model for the diagnosis of dyslexia has been associated with controversy: Under this approach, a dyslexia diagnosis requires that a discrepancy between recorded aptitude and documented achievement attain a criterial level. This model, introduced with the Individuals with Disabilities in Education Act (IDEA) in 1975, represented a standard until 2004 but is still followed in some areas. Shaywitz (136–137) critiques the requirement that an aptitude–achievement discrepancy appear at a criterial level for the identification of dyslexia; she observes that the model is founded on the notion that aptitude and achievement are typically correlated in an individual, and the presence of a marked discrepancy between the two suggests the presence of an unexpected challenge among an array of assets—a challenge that, like the reduction in reading skill that characterizes dyslexia, is circumscribed. An IQ measure is used to represent aptitude; Shaywitz points out, however, that the dyslexic individual's reduced reading experience may "artificially depress IQ scores" (135), and if a measured discrepancy between reading achievement and an (artificially depressed) IQ measure does not satisfy the criterion for a diagnosis of disability, a child will be denied treatment (131–132). Restori et al. point out, too, that young children are less likely to show an aptitude–achievement discrepancy that is wide enough to meet the criterial standard and will therefore be denied early intervention services, under a "wait-to-fail approach" to treatment (131). In addition, a child with below-average intellectual aptitude is unlikely to satisfy the discrepancy criterion and will not be served.

Shaywitz remarks that scientific advance in the understanding of dyslexia has permitted the development of more precise and powerful evaluation and diagnostic tools. It is that advance that we benefit from in the assessment of dyslexia, in the construction of the individual profile, and in the design of appropriate and effective treatment. Aptitude, achievement, and the transaction between the two are referenced under the current approach as we examine the balance of skills in the individual profile. Those skills include component skills in aptitude areas; assessment of component skills evaluates capacity to learn. Measured skills also include outcome skills or achievements, which represent what has been learned. The dynamic among the various skills invests the profile complex with its unique character, which will inform future planning.

The Assessment of Dyslexia

At seven years, eleven months and in the second grade, Hayden was assessed to determine the status of written-language development; his written-language profile, illumined through evaluation, indicated vulnerability both in outcome achievement performances and in component aptitudes measures. The contours of that profile—the patterning of assets and challenges, of score parities and divergences—suggested dyslexia, and that diagnosis led, crucially, to an apt recommendation for treatment. At nine years, nine months and in the fourth grade, Hayden was assessed on the same battery; the consequent profile resembled the first profile in fundamental skill balances but differed in critical outcome skill levels. Hayden had benefited from effective and successful written-language therapy, a result that also confirmed the appropriateness of the diagnosis.

The score sets created for this study are invented samples; Hayden is an invented personage. These two sample written-language score sets, however, resemble those in authentic assessment results, and the clinical questions raised by these created results are, likewise, quite real. The persistence and specificity of written-language challenge and of its underlying neural contingencies are fundamental to the definition and understanding of dyslexia; the insight that reading is hard because speech is easy (Liberman, *Speech* 427) has led to myriad research findings regarding the etiology, identification, and treatment of written-language challenge.

Established as fundamental to the activation of the alphabetic principle for reading and spelling and as foundational in the achievement of reading and writing fluency, phonological processing has been identified as the core deficit area in dyslexia. That deficit, in turn, has a neural reflex that is universal (Dehaene 244). That neural reflex involves underactivation in the area of the brain's letterbox area—the visual word form area in the brain's left occipitotemporal region that serves as a circuitry hub (Seidenberg 202), directing orthographic (print) stimuli toward sound and meaning interpretations—and in left posterior (back) circuitry areas. That underactivation, in the case of phonological processing deficit and dyslexia, accompanies hyperactivation in other (frontal) areas, a reflection of compensatory, inefficient circuitry in the dyslexic reader.

Assessment registers the consequences of neurological difference; remediation redresses the ramifications. As research advances our understanding of written-language challenge, treatment programs build on scientific findings and clinical insights to help children read and write. Scientific research and clinical experience indicate that programs featuring an explicit, code-based approach are most successful in guiding the student toward reading and spelling accuracy and fluency: At the locus where neurology does not serve the learner, instruction enters. A phonological processing deficit renders the written-language code opaque to the dyslexic learner; treatment therefore adopts a code-based approach under which phonemic segmentation and phoneme blending are trained directly, as are sound–symbol correspondences, word attack strategies, and orthographic conventions. In a highly structured and systematic program, Hayden was trained in the alphabetic code through direct instruction and focused practice; programs like the one that helped Hayden will feature a spiraling instructional design. Skill acquisition is regularly reinforced through multisensory (visual, auditory, and kinaesthetic) activation and reactivation of print–sound connections and through regular review of prior knowledge.

Scientific and clinical expertise informs design in the many thoughtful, effective programs based on these principles. Orton–Gillingham and derivative programs utilize rigorous program-design features to treat students who display dyslexia's core phonological processing deficit; Lindamood-Bell LiPS helps students whose phonemic processing challenges are particularly obdurate (Lindamood and Lindamood). RAVE-O (Wolf) is a powerful program for learners in the second through the fifth grade who would benefit from a special focus on orthographic processing and fluency. The most effective antidote to reading challenge is reading; in the face of reading challenge, the best route to a reading skill level that permits persistent reading is persistent treatment.

The battery of testing instruments presented here draws on clinical observations regarding test structure and efficacy. Just as there are many thoughtfully designed and effective research-based programs that have been developed and refined to address the treatment of dyslexia, numerous assessment instruments share key features with those included in the battery described here. The instruments in this battery are selected for the caliber and usefulness of the results they elicit; other well-designed assessment instruments might be utilized to measure the aptitudes and achievements that interact when an individual engages in literacy activities. Most important, in dyslexia assessment, is the inclusion of the crucial range of component-skill and outcome-skill measures, the close inspection of the individual written-language profile, the consultation of research findings to illuminate the significance of profile contours, a respect for the detail of student responses, and an appreciation of the power and promise of intervention. Careful, considered assessment, elucidating the rich and idiosyncratic individual profile of liabilities and gifts, and yielding questions as well as answers, speaks to that promise.

Works Cited

Adams, Marilyn Jager. "The Relation Between Alphabetic Basics, Word Recognition, and Reading." *What Research Has to Say About Reading Instruction.* Eds. S. Jay Samuels and Alan E. Farstrup. Newark, DE: International Reading Association, 2011. 4–24.

Dehaene, Stanislas. *Reading in the Brain.* New York: Penguin, 2009.

Ehri, Linnea. "Learning to Read Words." *Scientific Studies of Reading* 9:2 (2005): 167–188.

Gough, Philip B., and William E. Tunmer. "Decoding, Reading, and Reading Disability." *Remedial and Special Education* 7:1 (1986): 6–10.

Liberman, Alvin. *Speech: A Special Code.* Cambridge, MA: MIT Press, 1996.

Lindamood, Patricia, and Phyllis Lindamood. *Lindamood Phoneme Sequencing Program (LiPS).* Austin, TX: Pro-Ed, 1998.

Lyon, G. Reid, Sally E. Shaywitz, and Bennett A. Shaywitz. "A Definition of Dyslexia." *Annals of Dyslexia* 53:1 (2003): 1–14.

Melby-Lervag, Monica, Thomas S. Redick, and Charles Hulme. "Working Memory Training Does Not Improve Performance on Measure of Intelligence or Other Measures of 'Far Transfer': Evidence from a Meta-Analytic Review." *Perspectives on Psychological Science* 11:4 (2016): 512–534.

Moats, Louisa Cooke. *Spelling: Development, Disability, and Instruction.* Timonium, MD: York Press, 1995.

Morais, José, and Philippe Mousty. "The Causes of Phonemic Awareness." *Analytic Approaches to Human Cognition.* Eds. Jesus Alegria, Daniel Holender, José Junça de Morais, and Monique Radeau. Amsterdam: Elsevier Science Publishers, 1992. 193–212.

Restori, Albert F., Gary S. Katz, and Howard B. Lee. "A Critique of the IQ/Achievement Discrepancy Model for Identifying Specific Learning Disabilities." *Europe's Journal of Psychology* 5:4 (November 2009): 128–145.

Seidenberg, Mark. *Language at the Speed of Sight.* New York: Basic Books, 2017.

Shaywitz, Sally. *Overcoming Dyslexia.* New York: Vintage Books, 2005.

Vellutino, Frank R., and Jack M. Fletcher. "Developmental Dyslexia." *The Science of Reading: A Handbook.* Eds. Margaret J. Snowling and Charles Hulme. Oxford: Blackwell Publishing, 2009. 362–378.

Wolf, Maryanne. *The RAVE-O Program.* Longview, CO: Cambium/Sopris Learning, 2010.

Wolf, Maryanne, Alyssa Goldberg O'Rourke, Calvin Gidney, Maureen Lovett, Paul Cirino, and Robin Morris. "The Second Deficit: An Investigation of the Independence of Phonological and Naming-Speed Deficits in Developmental Dyslexia." *Reading and Writing: An Interdisciplinary Journal* 15 (2002): 43–72.

4 The Treatment of Dyslexia

Next Steps

Central to research on dyslexia and to clinical advances in its assessment, diagnosis, and treatment has been the insight that individuals who are challenged in reading and spelling achievement are confounded in their pursuit of basic literacy skills by a deficit in phonological awareness. Unable to conceptualize the structure of spoken words at the level of the phoneme, the minimal sound unit of spoken language, dyslexic individuals struggle to break down the speech stream into the phonemes that correspond to the letter or letter-cluster units (graphemes) from which written words are built. Those individuals are therefore unable to apply the alphabetic principle—the principle that the graphemes of written language map onto phonemes of our spoken language such that written spellings systematically represent spoken words—and cannot learn the phonics conventions, the set of sound–symbol correspondences that must be referenced for successful decoding and encoding. Instead, dyslexic individuals stand at the door to literacy without access to the key to the alphabetic code: phonemic awareness.

That phonemic awareness is the key by which the alphabetic code is accessed was explained lucidly, we saw, by Alvin Liberman in his comment that reading is hard because speech is easy (427). Liberman's insight derives from his deep understanding of the relation between spoken and written language: Written language is a second-order language modality, an invented tool that is founded on the spoken language but cannot be processed as speech is processed. As we read, we utilize the cortical sites and pathways that were designed for the apprehension of spoken language; neural architecture has been repurposed for the processing of print stimuli. We bring innate preparedness to spoken-language acquisition: We are prewired to learn to speak without effort. Biology has not prepared us, however, for the mastery of the written form. A few young children achieve literacy effortlessly, many become readers and writers with some effort, and a few need to invest a great deal of effort to attain phonemic awareness and then apply that acquired sensitivity to unlock the code of print.

The insight that we do not need phonemic awareness to process speech, because the production and apprehension of speech are precognitive processes, is due to Alvin Liberman; the underlying scientific contingencies and their consequences were investigated by his team at the Haskins Laboratories. The opacity of the phoneme in spoken language that has been revealed and illuminated in research on speech processing can be attributed to the efficiency and efficacy priorities in human language: To speak and listen as rapidly as we think means that we must speak and parse the speech signal much more rapidly than would be possible in a phoneme-by-phoneme processing of the speech stream. Instead, speaking and listening processes proceed by a different pulse, that of the syllable, in which the pertinent phonemes are coarticulated—formed in a shared gesture and merged for express packaging. It is to another Liberman, however, that we owe our understanding of the developmental particulars of the achievement of phonemic awareness and the impact of that development on the trajectory of early literacy growth. Alvin Liberman was married to Isabelle Liberman, whose scholarship in reading disability was seminal both in the investigation of the role of phonemic awareness in early reading and writing, and in the recognition of the significance of a core phonological processing deficit in dyslexia. Isabelle Liberman tested young children on their awareness of sublexical sound units—the constituent sound units within a word—by observing the children's capacity to count out phonemes in familiar monosyllabic words and to count out syllables in multisyllabic words (Liberman and Shankweiler). The four-year-olds did not count out phonemes accurately, but 50 percent of them arrived at accurate syllable counts. Among five-year-olds, more than 50 percent counted out syllables accurately, but fewer children—less than 20 percent—counted phonemes accurately. After completing their first school year, 90 percent of children counted syllables successfully; only 70 percent, however, successfully counted out phonemes. Liberman and Shankweiler conclude that phonemic segmentation is more challenging than is syllabic segmentation for young children, and that if phonemic segmentation skill does develop, it appears later than does syllabic segmentation ability. After a year of school, 10 percent of six-year-olds had not achieved syllabic segmentation; 30 percent still had not mastered the segmentation of spoken words at the phonemic level.

The developmental insights at which Liberman and Shankweiler arrived were significant in 1985 and remain so. They go on to explore causality: Is there a causal relationship between the metalinguistic awareness displayed by the capacity to count sublexical phonological units, on one hand, and, on the other hand, later literacy success? Liberman and Shankweiler discuss the pair of experiments carried out by Bradley and Bryant. After observing high correlations between phonological awareness levels in four- and five-year-olds and those children's later reading and spelling performance levels, Bradley and Bryant designed a training study: Children who had demonstrated lower phonological awareness in the first study were divided into four groups. One group received training on the identification of phoneme positions in CVC (consonant–vowel–consonant) words; a second group received the same phonological training and was also instructed on the representation of a syllable's phoneme sequence by means of alphabet letters. A third group was instructed as well, but the instructional focus was the semantics of the words rather than their phonology; a fourth group was the control group and received no instruction. Results indicated differential effects of training—the presence of training and the type of that training—on reading and spelling performance: Children who received training outperformed those who did not, children who received phonological training outperformed those who received semantic training, and children receiving alphabet-letter as well as phonological training outperformed those who received only phonological training, with a special benefit observed in spelling success.

The results reported by Bradley and Bryant are important because they demonstrate not only that component-skill level in phonological awareness predicts reading- and spelling-outcome performance but also that targeted enhancement of phonological awareness will result in improved outcome performance, suggesting a direct causal link between phonological awareness and reading and spelling success. Equally significant, too, is the evidence that phonological awareness can be developed through direct instruction—and that enrichment of that instruction with training on the application of letter–sound associations can enhance the effect of the training on literacy outcomes. The careful and inspired investigations, over decades and across disciplines, of scholars like Alvin Liberman, Isabelle Liberman, Donald Shankweiler, Lynette Bradley, and Peter Bryant provide findings that guide us in the assessment and diagnosis of dyslexia and then inform our plans for treatment.

And fundamental, in planning treatment, are the insights that metalinguistic knowledge can be taught and that metalinguistic awareness can be trained. As we saw earlier, *metalinguistic* behaviors are behaviors in which we objectify language. When we engage in metalinguistic behavior, we use language to reflect on, analyze, and discuss language objects: discourses, sentences, words, syllables, and phonemes. Natural spoken language, as we have seen, does not require our explicit awareness of its structure; ignoring its structural elements, we can utilize it efficiently and effectively to share our thoughts with one another. Given the rate at which we must speak and listen in order to exchange our thoughts in real time, we could never notice each phoneme. Because we are not prewired to notice phonemes explicitly, written language, which requires explicit awareness at the phonemic level, requires a degree of metalinguistic insight for its achievement, and this requirement is a liability for those for whom the phonemic insight represents a challenge. However, written language differs from spoken language not only in its prerequisite that knowledge of both written- and spoken-language structures be explicit rather than implicit but also in the way in which it is acquired. We are biologically prewired to acquire spoken language effortlessly; written language, however, is a cultural artifice whose conventions and processes are transmitted to a learner through study and training. Written language may be taught and often must be taught; it is learned with a modicum of effort, or with a fair degree of effort, or with a great amount of effort.

That instruction in written language not only is an option but also is a common requirement has been noted by educators, clinicians, and researchers; Mather and Wendling, for instance, observe that both written language and the phonological awareness that must be present in order for literacy learning to take place are teachable, that children with dyslexia must receive instruction that trains phonological awareness so that they can begin to learn to read and spell, and that the relation between phonological awareness growth and reading advances is reciprocal (135). Treatment for dyslexic learners—and there are many excellent and successful programs—is founded on the premise that, given systematic and deliberate program design, appropriate program selection, and persistent delivery of treatment, written language is learnable, as is phonemic awareness. And both written language and phonemic awareness, in the case of dyslexia, must be taught.

Treatment Programs

In Chapter 3, we considered Hayden's written-language profile, constructed after an evaluation of component and outcome skills. We first looked at the results of an evaluation completed when Hayden was in the fourth grade. Phonological processing challenge, reflected in *CTOPP-2* Phonological Awareness and Phonological Memory composite scores that were below the average range for age, was observed; single-word reading results on the *WRMT-III* Word Identification and Word Attack subtests, however, positioned Hayden in the average range for age, and *QRI-6* overall reading results showed that Hayden was instructional on grade-level text. Research has revealed, iteratively, that phonological processing skill is a prerequisite to reading success; a child must be able to segment language at the phonemic level in order to grasp the alphabetic principle governing written English, to learn and apply the set of phonics rules, and to decode familiar and unfamiliar words. How, then, could Hayden display age- and grade-appropriate reading levels, if phonological processing was an area of vulnerability? In an account of this anomaly, we observed that this evaluation in fact represented a reevaluation: Hayden was first evaluated in the second grade, when he was still struggling to break the alphabetic code and enter the world of literacy. In that first evaluation, Hayden's Phonological Awareness composite score was even lower, as were his single-word reading results and his overall reading level; decoding results were below the average range for age, and overall reading results indicated that Hayden was instructional at a text level below his assigned grade level. It was then revealed that a diagnosis of dyslexia following this first evaluation led to two years of Orton–Gillingham reading therapy; the fourth-grade evaluation results showed Hayden's positive response to treatment. Hayden's Phonological Awareness composite score, which reflected his ability not only to segment phonemes but also to perform phoneme manipulation operations, showed a slight uptick; two years of intensive and targeted therapy, however, permitted Hayden to advance his reading skills to a level such that the potential downward spiral of the Matthew effect was arrested. Consistent, nonetheless, with Hayden's reduced phonological processing skill was his spelling performance; challenged spelling, like challenged phonological processing skill, is characteristically a last, stubborn reminder of the presence of dyslexia.

Another reminder was the persistent split, on both evaluations, between listening comprehension level and decoding skill. On both evaluations, Hayden's performance on the *QRI-6* listening comprehension task revealed him to be instructional on text at a level two grades above his assigned grade level. Hayden's listening comprehension performance was not compromised, as were performances in other areas, by his dyslexia; because the texts were read to him, decoding demands were absent and therefore did not compromise his performance. On both evaluations, listening comprehension performance level represented a reading level Hayden might obtain if he were not constrained by phonological processing challenge: by dyslexia.

In Chapter 3, we also discussed the use of an aptitude–achievement discrepancy requirement for a dyslexia diagnosis (cf. Restori et al.). That tool has been discredited and has been discarded in many contexts; it can block early identification of dyslexia and early intervention efforts. Use of the aptitude–achievement discrepancy criterion vitiates appropriate diagnosis and intervention in cases in which it is less likely that the discrepancy will be observed at the criterial level. For instance, an adequate discrepancy is unlike to appear in the case of low intelligence; moreover, IQ—the aptitude measure—is often depressed when dyslexia has limited a child's reading activity. Although there are strong arguments against the use of a prescribed discrepancy level to define a diagnostic category, a discrepancy has clinical import. Hayden's score split between listening comprehension results and results on reading tasks calling on decoding, for instance, was an important clinical signal in the written-language profile of a student with strong linguistic comprehension aptitude that was not reflected in overall reading level. Hayden's single-word and overall reading performances attained age- and grade-appropriate levels on his second evaluation, yet his listening comprehension performance suggested unrealized reading potential.

This last observation suggests an ongoing therapy goal for Hayden: the full realization of his intellectual potential in academic pursuits. It suggests, too, that language comprehension is a special asset for Hayden; a treatment program in which that asset might be used to advantage would be a particularly appropriate choice. A program in which language is invoked in order to analyze language metalinguistically—in which language is used to teach, to explain, and to illuminate the writing system—would represent an apt match, given Hayden's written-language profile. The Orton–Gillingham program is such a program; among the various excellent treatments, Orton–Gillingham is well suited to a student with Hayden's array of challenges and strengths.

Orton–Gillingham

The Orton–Gillingham program, an evidence-based therapy program, was an early leader in the design of systematic, highly structured, and intensive treatments for dyslexia. Conceived as an individualized therapy regime, the approach has served as a model for many other effective programs (e.g., the Wilson Reading System) that may be administered to small groups of children. The Orton–Gillingham program instantiates the productive affiliation of scientific curiosity and clinical passion; Orton–Gillingham remediation was developed in the 1930s by Dr. Samuel Orton, a neurologist with a deep interest in learning disabilities, and Anna Gillingham, a psychologist. The program was founded, as has been its success, on the premise that dyslexia was rooted in a specific language-processing disorder. This perspective informed the structure and content of the treatment approach that became the Orton–Gillingham program.

Orton–Gillingham therapists are carefully trained, and lessons are structured deliberately both to accommodate individual challenge and progress and to conform consistently to key programmatic features: an explicit and code-based methodology, multisensory practice, sequential and controlled presentation of material, a spiraling and iterative rehearsal of learning, and an insistent emphasis on student success. The instructor assumes nothing, begins with basic concepts, builds on achievements, and systematically revisits prior learning. The insight that language-processing challenge leads to skill vacancies and knowledge gaps motivates a diagnostic-prescriptive methodology: The instructor persistently monitors student progress, adjusting lesson content to support the individual student's success. To reinforce skill development and buttress memory, the approach is multisensory: Skills are taught, activated, practiced, and reactivated in listening, speaking, reading, and writing exercises. Anna Gillingham and her collaborator, Bessie Stillman, explain their multisensory technique in terms of a "language triangle" (Gillingham and Stillman 40). The vertices of the language triangle represent three sensory processing modes—visual, auditory, and kinaesthetic—and the three sides of the triangle represent the types of associations that are strengthened when, for instance, a letter is read as a speech sound (auditory–visual association), when a letter form is copied in writing (visual–kinaesthetic association), and when a letter is written in response to a presented speech sound (kinaesthetic–auditory association). Multisensory learning is reinforced learning; the multisensory approach is also integrative. Responding to multiple learning and memory cues in written-language behaviors, the student also makes connections among reading, writing, speaking, and listening processes and products.

Phoneme segmentation is trained, and because the dyslexic student struggles to unlock the phonology–orthography code on which alphabetic reading and writing are based, Orton–Gillingham makes explicit that coding. Anna Gillingham devised a systematic sequence by which *phonograms* (the graphemes of English—the letters or letter clusters representing individual phonemes) would be taught. As these building blocks of the written-language system are established, the student learns the connections that constitute the phonics system of written English. Training in that phonics system—in the set of sound–symbol associations and their application to reading and to spelling—is deliberate. Assuming neither that the dyslexic learner will acquire phonics knowledge spontaneously nor that the learner will spontaneously apply that knowledge, the phonics instructor is fully explicit. In the typical elementary classroom, different approaches to phonics instruction—instruction in letter–sound relationships and in their application to literacy activities—may be selected. Under the incidental (or *analytic*) phonics approach, whole words are introduced before phonics learning is established; children are encouraged to deduce letter–sound relationships, analyzing a familiar word to identify sound–letter associations and then applying those phonics insights to an unfamiliar word. Under the explicit (or *synthetic*) approach, in contrast, words are synthesized or built up from known parts; in this explicit approach, the sound–symbol associations are introduced first. Grapheme–phoneme correspondences, made explicit, are taught before sounds are blended to form syllables or whole words. In the Orton–Gillingham system, phonics instruction is fully explicit.

The commitment in Orton–Gillingham programming to explicit instruction accompanies and supports a broader commitment to student success. Aware that dyslexic children are vulnerable to experiences of academic failure, the instructor is dedicated to their successful achievement in every lesson, and the program is designed to ensure that success. Design features that support student success include *controlled presentation* and *spiraling methodology*. Under a controlled presentation of content and processes, the student is never asked to produce a behavior that has not been taught explicitly. The predesigned sequencing helps to prevent the appearance in the lesson plan of items on which the student has not been trained; in addition, the instructor utilizes controlled stimuli. Each lesson, for instance, includes a segment in which the student reads connected text; here, the instructor will select controlled text—orthographically regular text on which the student will encounter only those orthographic patterns, apply only those sound–symbol associations, and consult only those conventions of print that have been taught and are now familiar. A spiraling methodology is one in which learning is revisited regularly. After a topic, an association, a generalization, or a skill is introduced, it reappears systematically. A student first develops basic concept knowledge or a basic skill; when a concept is reactivated or a skill is reviewed in the context of new learning, that knowledge becomes both more deep and more deeply established. An opportunity to display the pretrained skill, moreover, is an opportunity for the student to succeed.

The concepts and skills that are taught in the Orton–Gillingham system are ordered, proceeding from the most fundamental practice to the more complex generalizations. Meeting two or three times per week in one-hour sessions, the instructor and the student advance through an instructional sequence that begins with training in phoneme awareness, letter names, and associated letter sounds. Systematically, the student amasses knowledge of predictable sound–symbol phonics relationships, studying the consonants, the short vowels, the consonant *digraphs* (consonant letter pairs, such as *th* or *ch* or *sh*, that are associated with single sounds), and the consonant *blends* (consonant letter pairs, such as *bl* or *tr* or *st*, that are associated with two distinct sounds in sequence). Next, conditional or variant orthographic patterns are studied: vowel letter pairs (such as *ai* or *oa*) or patterns (such as a long vowel in a word ending with a silent *e*), consonant letter clusters whose occurrence is governed by position in a word (such as *ch ~ tch* or *j ~ dge*), hard and soft *c* and *g*, and vowel cluster variants whose occurrence is governed by position (such as *oi ~ oy* or *ai ~ ay*). The student studies spelling generalizations, such as the rule whereby *f*, *l*, *s*, and *z*, when following a short vowel sound, are doubled at the end of a monosyllabic word. The student next learns six different syllable patterns commonly occurring in English and studies syllabication rules. In addition, the student learns spelling patterns for suffixes (such as *-ed* or *-tion*) that represent instances in the morphophonemic orthography of English in which morphology (word structure) rather than phonology (sound structure) governs spelling. The student also learns spelling rules that apply when a suffix is added to an English content word and goes on to study Latin-based roots and affixes (as in *predict, receive,* and *transportation*) and Greek combining forms (as in *telescope* and *geology*).

Progressing through this carefully arranged curriculum, the student not only assembles knowledge about the structure of the written language but also practices the Orton–Gillingham approach: A daunting task can be broken down into manageable and sequenced components and mastered through systematic activation, reactivation, and internalization of knowledge and skills. This skill practice represents the heart of Orton–Gillingham treatment; systematic practice occurs in every lesson.

Just as the Orton–Gillingham methodology and curriculum are highly structured, the lesson itself is organized so that the learning events follow a sequence that is predictable and comprehensive. Each lesson offers the student opportunities to read and to write; the lesson also invites the student to work at the subword level and then at the level of the word, the sentence, and the text. And in each lesson, the student activates learning through auditory–visual, visual–kinaesthetic, and kinaesthetic–auditory connections. A model lesson typically has four sections; the first section (about ten minutes) includes review of learned phonograms, a brief blending practice in which the student blends sounds in a series of invented syllables, and explicit instruction on a new pattern or concept. In the second section (again, about ten minutes), the student reads words and sentences in which the new concept or pattern appears. In the third section (perhaps twenty minutes), the student writes. At the sound level, the writing involves a reversed phonogram practice in which the instructor presents a sound and the student writes the associated phonogram. At the word level, the student spells items, using *simultaneous oral spelling*: The student repeats the target word, sounds out the word while tapping for each phoneme, writes the word while naming each letter, and then reads the word. In a dictation exercise at the end of the third section, the student applies the lesson's new learning and integrates it with prior knowledge in order to write a dictated sentence. In the fourth section of the lesson, the student spends fifteen to twenty minutes reading text. Materials in all of the sections are controlled: The student is never asked to apply concepts that have not been studied or to demonstrate skills that have not been practiced.

The legacies of Dr. Samuel Orton, of Anna Gillingham, and of the Orton–Gillingham treatment program are vast. Grounded in science, featuring pedagogy that is informed by deep clinical sensitivity, deliberately designed, the program has served—in design, approach, and content—as a model for an array of derivative programs. The availability of diverse treatment options permits the parent, the school system, and the evaluator to seek a therapeutic program that best suits the individual dyslexic learner. Orton–Gillingham treatment is a strong choice for many children; the prescribed structure and a curriculum that permits the advancing student to study written English in systematic detail benefit the learner who struggles with specific, unexpected reading challenge. Orton–Gillingham is especially appropriate for a student for whom academic study and content learning are appealing—for a student who, like Hayden, displays a special strength in linguistic comprehension.

The Orton–Gillingham program incorporates phonemic awareness training in its lessons; in activities like simultaneous oral spelling, for instance, the student taps out the phonemes in a word and then retrieves the letters associated with that phoneme string. And the instructor, sensitive to individual student need, will incorporate further phoneme segmentation practice when indicated. Some students, however, encounter a more profound challenge in phonological processing and require more intensive and extensive work to learn to segment the speech stream into phonemes. For this type of student, Lindamood–Bell LiPS is often recommended.

Lindamood–Bell LiPS

In 1986, Nanci Bell, an educator, and Patricia Lindamood, a speech pathologist, founded Lindamood–Bell Learning Processes. The company has developed a number of programs; of these, the Lindamood Phoneme

Sequencing Program for Reading, Spelling, and Speech (LiPS) addresses the phonological processing, reading, and spelling challenges that accompany dyslexia (Lindamood and Lindamood). The LiPS therapy is typically a short-term, individualized, intensive treatment over a period of eight to twelve weeks; two to four hours of daily therapy are administered five days per week. The concentration and focus of programming are intentional design components. Like the Orton–Gillingham therapist, the LiPS instructor breaks down the passage to reading achievement into a series of concrete and manageable steps. The student builds on trained skills to achieve new learning; each skill is therefore taught to mastery, with instructional pace calibrated to the needs of the individual student. A spiraling practice design, as in Orton–Gillingham lessons, permits the student to revisit, review, and strengthen prior learning. And, as in the Orton–Gillingham model, instruction in phonemic awareness and in phonics conventions is systematic and explicit. Distinctive in the LiPS program, however, is its special emphasis on sensory learning.

Under the LiPS approach, therapy for emergent readers (in the kindergarten through the third grade) or for older dyslexic students begins with the establishment of phoneme awareness before sound–symbol associations are addressed: The identification and production of individual sounds will represent the initial therapeutic focus. The student first works on sound perception and then progresses to sound production; LiPS program instructors teach students to determine the identity, number, and order in a sequence of phonemes in word context. After working on phonemic awareness, students study sound–symbol associations and the application of new skills, such as the blending of sounds into words, to reading and spelling tasks. Through reading practices on connected text and supported writing, students advance to independent reading and writing. As in the Orton–Gillingham approach, students read controlled text.

The LiPS program, like Orton–Gillingham, uses a multisensory approach to instruction and practice. Focusing on sensorimotor awareness in the oral area, an instructor guides the student to hear, see, and feel the sounds of speech—to feel and label the vocal-tract movements of lips, tongue, and throat by discovering the lip, tongue, and mouth gestures that are used when specific sounds are produced. Guided by this kinaesthetic feedback, the student then learns to identify, enumerate, and order the sounds in words. Bell defines phonemic awareness as "the ability to perceive the identity, number, and order of sound within words ... the ability to hear sounds in words [and] segment one from the other" (25). Focusing on process, Bell characterizes phonemic awareness as a basic "sensory–cognitive" process underlying the integration of skills in reading (27).

Building sensory–cognitive learning into phonemic awareness training under LiPS involves a special focus on the articulatory feedback in the vocal mechanism: That feedback represents a *"concrete* way to perceive sounds" (Bell 34). Feedback via multiple sensory modalities permits the student to crosscheck sensory information; the instructor also uses phoneme labels as mnemonic supports. Many of these labels reference features indicating place and manner of articulation. For example, the bilabial stops /p/ and /b/ are *lip poppers*; the alveolar stops /t/ and /d/ are *tongue tappers*; the velar stops /k/ and /g/ are *tongue scrapers*; the labiodental fricatives /f/ and /v/ are *lip coolers*; the alveolar fricatives /s/ and /z/ are *skinny air*; the palatal fricatives /sh/ and /zh/ are *fat air*; the palatal affricates /ch/ and /j/ are *fat-puffy air*. The consonant sound examples listed here occur in voiced and unvoiced pairs, such that vocal cord vibration accompanies a voiced sound and no vibration accompanies an unvoiced sound. That feature difference is reflected in the labels used in LiPS instruction: *quiet* (for unvoiced sounds) and *noisy* (for voiced sounds). From a pedagogical perspective, these mnemonic labels that reference accessible articulatory gestures provide yet another way to invest abstract phonemic segments with concrete distinctiveness.

After consonant and vowel sounds have been explored, the student engages in *tracking*. In tracking, the student develops skill in phoneme sequencing, learning to utilize the sensory input from articulatory feedback to investigate the sound composition of a syllable. Students first use a sequence of tiles that depict the mouth in various articulatory positions; in a double-coding procedure, phonemes are associated both with pictures and with their mnemonic labels. Next, in another creative innovation that has since appeared in various forms in other programs and that concretizes the abstractions not only of the phoneme but also of phonemic sequencing, colored blocks are used for phonemic awareness training. Bell (35–36) explains this tracking practice: A set of small colored blocks is available for the representation of sounds within a syllable; the student responds to a syllable pattern such as *pim*, choosing one block to represent each sound in the syllable's three-sound sequence. The student tracks the phoneme sequence by touching each block and saying the sound it represents; uttering each sound, the student experiences sensory feedback in its articulation. When the student is asked to use the blocks to represent a phoneme substitution—to change *pim* to *fim*, for instance—the student will replace the pertinent block—in this case, the first block—with a differently colored block and will explain the change—stating, in this case, that "the lip popper went out and the lip cooler went in" (36). Bell states, "The labels reinforce the articulatory feedback … the student is feeling … The stimulation purposely begins with feeling" (36). This articulatory feedback makes the phoneme segments concrete; the phoneme labels, which reference that articulatory feedback, suggest imagery, another key Lindamood–Bell treatment component. Letter tiles are also used for tracking; the blocks, however, which lack letter tags and are distinguished only by color, allow the student to respond to the characteristics that distinguish phonemes in syllabic context: sameness/difference, number, and order. Asking the student to track with blocks, the instructor differentiates between segmentation when reading/spelling and segmentation that focuses on and solidifies phoneme awareness itself by concretizing the syllable's phonemic composition and sequence.

Lindamood–Bell's multisensory approach also includes an emphasis on imagery. Pertinent to the early literacy processes addressed in the LiPS program would be *symbol imagery*; Bell explains that symbol imagery involves "the ability to visualize letters in words. Seeing letters in the mind's eye is symbol imagery" (20). She explains that as spellers, when we hear the nonword *fip* pronounced, we visualize its spelling; if we are asked to change *fip* to *fap*, we watch, on our "imaged screen," the letter *i* disappear and the letter *a* appear (20–21). She explains further that strengths in symbol imagery, in phonemic awareness, and in spelling seem to correlate. Symbol imagery supports the development of phonemic awareness; it provides yet another way for the student to distinguish phoneme segments, discerning difference, number, and order.

In the Lindamood–Bell LiPS curriculum, the sensory component plays a major role. The student profits from multiple sources of sensory information, learns to use those types of input, and integrates them in literacy contexts. The Lindamood–Bell "*independence* paradigm" (Bell 33) begins with sensory input; the student, learning to self-monitor and self-correct by systematically utilizing the kinaesthetic, tactile, auditory, and visual sensory input incorporated in LiPS activities, will advance toward independence in reading and spelling. Sensory associations lend concreteness to the abstract objects of language, such as the phoneme; a phoneme may be made concrete both in a photograph of an associated oral gesture and through a mnemonic label. That "dual coding" (Bell 24) in sensory input is also a signal feature of the Lindamood–Bell approach.

The LiPS program shares with the Orton–Gillingham system the pedagogical features of a spiraling design, practice to mastery, and code-based and explicit training in phonemic awareness and sound–symbol associations. Both programs utilize multisensory practice; in Orton–Gillingham, that practice involves spelling and reading activities, whereas LiPS emphasizes the sensory input of speech movements. And this feature of the LiPS multisensory approach reflects a greater emphasis in the LiPS program on knowledge and skill growth through amassed sensory experience, whereas Orton–Gillingham focuses on the application, the review, and the reapplication of a growing knowledge base through direct instruction and directed skill rehearsal. In addition, the LiPS program emphasizes the development of "sensory–cognitive functions" (Bell 27) through a distinctive discovery approach in its pedagogy. Guided by the LiPS instructor in a discovery process, students gain sensory awareness that helps them build conceptual knowledge.

Both the LiPS instructor and the Orton–Gillingham therapist recognize the primacy of the phonological processing deficit in dyslexia; treatment targets the effects of that deficit. LiPS focuses more persistently on the development of phonemic awareness and is especially appropriate for the learner with profound challenge in this area. Another program, the RAVE-O program, also acknowledges the crucial role of the deficit in phonological processing that accompanies dyslexia; RAVE-O instruction, too, is code-based, explicit instruction in reading and writing. However, RAVE-O is designed to accommodate those dyslexic learners who would benefit from a special focus on orthographic processing and fluency.

RAVE-O

The RAVE-O reading intervention program was designed by Maryanne Wolf, a scholar and educator who directs the Center for Dyslexia, Diverse Learners, and Social Justice at UCLA and is the former director of the Center for Reading and Language Research at Tufts University. The RAVE-O—Retrieval, Automaticity, Vocabulary, Engagement with Language, and Orthography (Wolf et al., "The RAVE-O Intervention" 87)—program, like the Orton–Gillingham and Lindamood–Bell LiPS therapies, provides systematic intervention through code-based instruction. At the various levels of natural language (the phonology, the morphology, the lexicon, the syntax, and the semantics), implicit knowledge is made explicit. Direct instruction in the written-language areas of orthography and phonics establishes the firm knowledge bases on which children draw as they develop automatic application of the conventions of written language; engaging exercises stimulate learning and help children to draw connections across knowledge systems. It is through these connections that children achieve fluency in the integrative act of reading, and that fluency in reading and comprehending is focused in RAVE-O. Founded on and deeply grounded in research, the RAVE-O program offers a broad-based approach to reading fluency development; its activities are designed to build automaticity at the different spoken- and written-language levels pertinent to reading.

RAVE-O utilizes key pedagogical practices featured in the Orton–Gillingham and Lindamood–Bell LiPS methods. The spiraling instructional design evident in the Orton–Gillingham and Lindamood–Bell LiPS programs is utilized in the RAVE-O program as well; under an integrative approach, the RAVE-O instructor systematically revisits prior learning and invites students to make connections between new and prior learning. As in the Orton–Gillingham and LiPS programs, too, students are trained explicitly to activate learning in skill application; as in Lindamood–Bell LiPS, moreover, playful discovery is incorporated in the highly motivating program activities.

The story of RAVE-O is the story of decades of educational and neurological research (Wolf et al., "The RAVE-O Intervention" 84–85). Key research insights that anticipated the program's inception included Chall's observation that letter-name knowledge is an important predictor of later reading achievement (cf. Badian) and Geschwind's observation regarding a nineteenth-century alexia (acquired reading loss) case study in which both reading ability and color-naming capacity were lost. Noting that the character of reading breakdown depends on the site of neural disconnection, Geschwind proposed that reading and color naming share a neurological base; he suggested, further, that color-naming skill might be associated with reading preparedness. Following Geschwind's proposal, his student Martha Denckla tested dyslexic children; their color naming was accurate but slow (Denckla and Rudel). These findings stimulated Wolf's research on the predictive relationship between performance on rapid automatized naming (RAN) tasks and reading performance. In the RAN task, the student is asked to name items in a stimulus series—in a series of colors, objects, numbers, or letters—as quickly as possible.

As we saw earlier, Wolf and her colleagues investigated the possibility that phonological awareness and naming-speed performance each contribute unique variance to dyslexic children's performance on reading tasks and found that naming-speed measures made contributions beyond those of phonological processing measures to variance on word attack, word identification, and reading comprehension measures (Wolf et al., "The Second Deficit"). Although scholars such as Seidenberg take a "phonological umbrella" (Seidenberg 176) approach, concluding that "rapid naming processes would be best subsumed under the rubric of phonology" (Wolf et al., "The RAVE-O Intervention" 85), Wolf et al. conclude that "phoneme awareness and naming speed are ... the tips of at least two different but overlapping sources of reading breakdown" ("The RAVE-O Intervention" 85), recognizing the significance of the core phonological processing deficit but distinguishing a second and distinct dyslexia subtype. Aggregating research data, Wolf and her colleagues (85–86) propose a second dyslexia deficit: a naming-speed deficit that inhibits the development of reading fluency.

Wolf was motivated by these results to search for an intervention model that would address not only phonological processing challenge but also fluency and comprehension issues. That intervention would promote the development of high-quality representations at the various spoken- and written-language levels and would build automatic connections across those levels (Wolf et al., "The RAVE-O Intervention" 87). The RAVE-O program is "about teaching young readers to enrich and connect all their knowledge about a word as fast as possible" (87). When successful, the program has consequences that replicate, neurologically, the natural results of reading maturation (87). By enriching lexical knowledge, by refining the representations of linguistic elements, by training rapid orthographic recognition, and by strengthening the connections between linguistic and orthographic segments, the program builds fluency in children's responses to print through the automatic retrieval of associated language forms.

RAVE-O is designed for second- to fifth-grade learners. Working with small groups of children, the instructor dedicates a segment of the lesson to code-based training in reading and spelling; children receive explicit instruction in phoneme awareness and in sound–symbol phonics correspondences. Connections between the level of sound structure and the other levels of spoken and written language are emphasized in the activities that follow. In the RAVE-O portion of the lesson, orthographic processing and fluency are focused. The instructor seeks not only to establish explicit and high-quality representations for spoken- and written-language elements—in precise and complete phonological structures, in common orthographic patterns, in the orthographic representations of frequently occurring morphemes, and in well-defined semantic alternatives associated with a lexical or orthographic form—but also to build automatic connections among these elements when they are represented in text.

Orthographic training features an emphasis on the rapid recognition of common orthographic patterns to promote automaticity, with computer games and manipulatives utilized to engage learners and promote multimodal, multisensory learning. The spiraling design in the lesson sequence permits multiple exposures to orthographic shapes in words and in letter patterns, solidifying learning. Of special interest is the extension of the explicit instruction that characterizes phonological awareness and phonics training to those aspects of morphology that are reflected in the morphophonemic orthography of English. We observed earlier that the morphophonemic orthography of English references both sound- and word-structure segments; this insight is reflected in the RAVE-O curriculum in its instruction on suffixes, for instance, which are given the mnemonic label "Ender Benders" (88), referencing the way in which a suffix inflects root meaning or derives new meaning: The knowledge implicit in spoken-language use is made explicit for the reader/speller. The same type of attention is directed toward syntactic abstractions such as grammatical categories; as in the case of morphology, the implicit knowledge of phrasal and sentence forms that children utilize in spoken language is made explicit for them so that it can be applied in reading and writing contexts.

The RAVE-O program also places special focus on the lexicon, an area that, as we saw earlier, is involved in critical transaction with reading growth; Stanovich indicates the consequences of the Matthew effect in the bidirectional relationship between vocabulary knowledge and reading growth in the advancing reader. Children receive a weekly set of *core words*; the words in that set feature phonemes studied in the first part of the lesson. The core words also display a featured orthographic pattern; in addition, the set includes words associated with multiple meanings. The core words represent exemplars through which the instructor can demonstrate the language function of the various spoken- and written-language levels that are consulted in the integrative act of reading. RAVE-O activities enrich lexical knowledge about terms in the core word set, helping students understand, for instance, how connotation deepens lexical meaning or how position in a semantic network adds precision to the individual entry. Images are used here as mnemonic devices.

In the end, the goal of reading treatment is the gift of reading itself: reading for the story, for knowledge, for love of reading. That gift arrives in fluent comprehension, which in turn depends on automatic and accurate decoding: on reading fluency. Fluent, lucid reading of connected text is emphasized in the series of stories planned for each week of treatment; students activate prior learning in repeated—timed and untimed—readings of the week's Minute Stories. Core words for the week appear in the stories in ways that call attention to the multiple semantic possibilities of a particular orthographic string, and repeated readings allow the student to revisit learning associated with the week's orthographic and morphological lessons. After reading the text, the learner applies RAVE-O's Think Thrice strategies: Think Ahead! Think Back! Think for Yourself! Enjoined to predict and to monitor for comprehension, the reader is also urged to look inward. The invitation in the third Think Thrice strategy epitomizes the program's respect for the individual student and the focus on student engagement.

The emphasis on engagement, referenced in the program's full title, reflects the programmatic choice to "incorporate an additional system ... the affective–motivational one" (Wolf et al., "The RAVE-O Intervention" 89). The excitement generated in the RAVE-O classroom reflects an intentional feature of the pedagogy: The child's affective–motivational system is deliberately invoked, because it is instrumental in learning and in progress toward automaticity (89). The practices and the content features of the program are motivating and are memorable to children; their intrinsic appeal promotes the learning that is crucial to reading growth. They also promote engagement in reading; as we have seen, the Matthew effect in reading is countered by persistent, engaged reading of text. In the attractive detail of its programming and in its overall design, RAVE-O advances students toward literacy. The focus on student success that has appeared in each of the three programs we have considered—Orton–Gillingham, Lindamood–Bell LiPS, and RAVE-O—reflects attention in all three programs to best teaching practices: an awareness of the critical roles of motivation, inspiration, and engagement in effective instruction. In the RAVE-O program, the commitment to student success extends beyond careful curricular design and controlled presentation of content; it is reflected in captivating materials, creative activities, and a recognition of the power of joyful learning.

As a research- and evidence-based program, RAVE-O shows a special strength in the scientific documentation of its efficacy. For a decade, the program was assessed against other models in randomized treatment–control studies; results showed students who had received RAVE-O treatment outperforming children receiving other treatments on word attack, word identification, textual reading, and comprehension measures (Wolf et al., "The RAVE-O Intervention" 89–90). Of particular interest is the superior performance of students in the RAVE-O treatment group when vocabulary and fluent comprehension were assessed; both skill areas are notably resistant to intervention (90). Wolf et al. emphasize the significance of vocabulary growth to rapid retrieval and to comprehension growth, the ultimate goal in RAVE-O training (89).

We see that the RAVE-O program, like the Orton–Gillingham system and the Lindamood–Bell LiPS approach, addresses the phonological processing deficit in dyslexia through code-based and explicit reading and writing instruction. Like Orton–Gillingham and LiPS, RAVE-O ensures that students experience success systematically through careful activity design, controlled presentation of content, and controlled text. As in the other two programs, a spiraling instructional design helps students to renew associations in learned material and establish connections between prior knowledge and new learning. Like Lindamood–Bell LiPS, RAVE-O invites students to engage in discovery. RAVE-O's special emphasis on student engagement, its deep research base, and its strong efficacy documentation are distinctive; distinctive, too, is its programmatic focus on orthographic processing, automaticity, and fluency. It represents an especially appropriate treatment choice, therefore, for the dysfluent reader.

Treatment

We have considered three well-known and influential treatment programs for the dyslexic learner. In overall focus and in the detail of treatment, each program is informed by research; all three programs address the phonological processing deficit associated with dyslexia, and each incorporates best clinical and pedagogical practices in order to bring the dyslexic learner into literacy. The three programs share important design features: a highly structured and systematic approach, a multisensory and multimodal learning experience, and explicit and code-based training. Direct instruction in the conventions of written language accompanies a structured, sequential, and cumulative curriculum that progresses from basic to more complex content; a spiraling pedagogy permits students to revisit and reactivate prior learning and to draw connections between prior knowledge and new concepts. Controlled presentation of material and controlled text help to ensure consistent and persistent student success in an arena—the world of literacy—in which the dyslexic student has so often failed.

In each program, distinctive facets of treatment are emphasized—sensory–cognitive learning, for instance, in the LiPS program, or attention to the affective–motivational system in RAVE-O. Significantly, each program is associated with a special treatment focus. The Orton–Gillingham program, with its careful structure and a curriculum that progresses systematically through the written English system, is particularly appropriate for the learner who is confronted by unexpected and circumscribed challenge in reading and spelling. A student with a strength in linguistic comprehension can draw on that capacity as the conventions of the written language are introduced, rehearsed, applied, and revisited. The Lindamood–Bell LiPS program, with its emphasis on sensory learning, would be a good choice for a student who enjoys learning through the sensory modality. The emphasis, in LiPS, on the development of phonemic awareness makes that program a strong choice for the learner who needs intensive work in this area before basic reading and spelling conventions can begin to make sense. RAVE-O, typically administered in a small learning group, is distinguished by its emphasis on orthographic processing and fluency. RAVE-O would be an apt choice for the child who may decode accurately but reads dysfluently.

Each program addresses phonological processing and the phonology–orthography interface—the alphabetic principle on which the English writing system is based—through direct training in phoneme segmentation and explicit instruction in the alphabetic code. Each program, in its own systematic way, uses spoken language to make explicit the principles of natural language and to teach the conventions of the written language. Each profits from decades of research initiatives revealing that, although reading is hard because speech is easy (Liberman 427), reading can develop through explicit training, as can awareness of the phonemic structure of natural language. Spoken language, moreover, can be recruited for the metalinguistic investigation that yields an explicit understanding of language structures. Reading and writing can be taught and, for the dyslexic learner, must be taught.

Works Cited

Badian, Nathlie. "Predicting Reading Ability over the Long Term: The Changing Roles of Letter Naming, Phonological Awareness, and Orthographic Processing." *Annals of Dyslexia* 45 (1995): 79–96.

Bell, Nanci. *Seeing Stars*. San Luis Obispo: Gander Publishing, 1997.

Bradley, Lynette, and Peter E. Bryant. "Categorizing Sounds and Learning to Read: A Causal Connection." *Nature* 301 (February 1983): 419–421.

Chall, Jeanne. *Stages of Reading Development*. New York: McGraw-Hill, 1983.

Denckla, Martha Bridge, and Rita G. Rudel. "Rapid Automatized Naming (RAN): Dyslexia Differentiated from Other Learning Disabilities." *Neuropsychologia* 14 (1976): 471–479.

Geschwind, Norman. *Selected Papers on Language and the Brain*. Dordrecht: D. Reidel, 1974.

Gillingham, Anna, and Bessie Stillman. *Remedial Training for Children with Specific Disability in Reading, Spelling, and Penmanship*. Cambridge, MA: Educators Publishing Service, 1995.

Liberman, Alvin. *Speech: A Special Code*. Cambridge, MA: MIT Press, 1996.

Liberman, Isabelle Y., and Donald Shankweiler. "Phonology and the Problems of Learning to Read and Write." *Remedial and Special Education* 6 (1985): 8–17.

Lindamood, Patricia, and Phyllis Lindamood. *Lindamood Phoneme Sequencing Program (LiPS)*. Austin, TX: Pro-Ed, 1998.

Mather, Nancy, and Barbara J. Wendling. *Essentials of Dyslexia Assessment and Intervention*. Hoboken, NJ: John Wiley & Sons, 2012.

Restori, Albert F., Gary S. Katz, and Howard B. Lee. "A Critique of the IQ/Achievement Discrepancy Model for Identifying Specific Learning Disabilities." *Europe's Journal of Psychology* 5:4 (November 2009): 128–145.

Seidenberg, Mark. *Language at the Speed of Sight*. New York: Basic Books, 2017.

Stanovich, Keith. "Matthew Effects in Reading: Some Consequences of Individual Differences in the Acquisition of Literacy." *Reading Research Quarterly* 21:4 (Fall 1986): 360–407.

Wolf, Maryanne. *The RAVE-O Program.* Longview, CO: Cambium/Sopris Learning, 2010.

Wolf, Maryanne, Alyssa Goldberg O'Rourke, Calvin Gidney, Maureen Lovett, Paul Cirino, and Robin Morris. "The Second Deficit: An Investigation of the Independence of Phonological and Naming-Speed Deficits in Developmental Dyslexia." *Reading and Writing: An Interdisciplinary Journal* 15 (2002): 43–72.

Wolf, Maryanne, Mirit Barzillai, Stephanie Gottwald, Lynne Miller, Kathleen Spencer, Elizabeth Norton, Maureen Lovett, and Robin Morris. "The RAVE-O Intervention: Connecting Neuroscience to the Classroom." *Mind, Brain, and Education* 3:2 (2009): 84–93.

5 The Dyslexic Writer

Reading and Writing

Alvin Liberman's observation that reading is hard because speech is easy is both confirmatory and explanatory. A fundamental challenge of literacy is explained: Speech is easy because we can ignore a language level that we are not prepared, biologically, to access: the level of the phonological abstraction of the phoneme. Reading is hard, however, because we cannot ignore that abstract level when we read and write: We must segment the speech stream phonemically in order to process print. And the distinctive and circumscribed character of dyslexia, a challenge that inhibits achievement in the cultural convention of literacy, is confirmed: The core capacity that distinguishes the successful from the challenged reader/writer is neither a general ability nor a natural, evolved capacity. Access to the phonemic level is not requisite to the processing of natural language; we are not prewired to parse the speech stream at the phonemic level. Reading is hard because speech is easy, and writing is often harder than reading.

And for the dyslexic reader, writing may be much more difficult than reading. We observed that on Hayden's written-language evaluations, his spelling performance on the *TWS-5*, below the average range for age when he was first assessed at seven years, eleven months, remained below that average range when he was assessed two years later. At that second testing point, Hayden had received Orton–Gillingham treatment, and his performances on single-word reading measures—*WRMT-III* Word Identification and Word Attack—had advanced to the average range; in spite of substantive reading growth, however, Hayden's spelling challenge persisted. We noted aspects of spelling that contribute to its challenge: Spelling requires full accuracy, and mastery of the sound-to-print mapping required by spelling is more elusive than is that of the print-to-sound mapping in successful decoding. Spelling, cited in the IDA's definition of dyslexia, is a profound challenge for the dyslexic student; more broadly, the challenged dyslexic speller is the challenged dyslexic writer. Written composition, at its many levels—the writing process, at its many stages—presents signature difficulty for the dyslexic student. Shaywitz comments on the unrelenting character of dyslexia's writing issues:

> In addition to problems with poor reading, poor spelling is often a sign of dyslexia ... As a child who is dyslexic goes on in school, difficulties with spelling persist. In fact, spelling errors may remain long after a dyslexic child or adult has learned to decode most words accurately ... Children who are dyslexic frequently have abominable handwriting.
>
> (Shaywitz 114)

The *transcription* skills of writing—handwriting and spelling—stand out as special areas of vulnerability for the dyslexic writer; Shaywitz remarks, too, that "composition ... is challenging for the dyslexic reader" (254). Shaywitz's observations are consonant with those of other researchers, educators, and clinicians in the field of dyslexia.

In order to treat the dyslexic learner, we need to appreciate the great challenge faced by that learner when encountering the concurrent and multilevel demands of written text production. The consequences of that challenge are evident; in order to design effective intervention, however, we must not only observe the magnitude of its outcome—the performance deficit evinced in the written product—but also understand the character of and interactions among the lower-level (transcription) capacities and the upper-level (composition) performance. To explore that dynamic and appreciate the dyslexic writer's experience during the writing process, we first consider the writing process itself. Deeply connected in dyslexia, reading and writing are connected, too, in the typical developmental trajectory. A review of scholarship on the reading–writing relationship and of research into the functional and neurological detail of the writing process yields the insight that spelling challenge has a unique and pernicious impact on writing: on writing procedures, development, and output. That insight also informs treatment design: The skill elements in the multilayer dynamic of the writing process, diverse and distinct, are interconnected, as are the transactions—both concurrent and sequential—among them. Those skills and transactions contribute together to the writing outcome; accurate diagnosis that not only observes the face of writing challenge but also identifies its sources—componential, transactional—is paramount.

Writing and Reading

We have observed the transactions among constructs, behaviors, and skills that would be situated at the various interstices in a model of written language. Growth in phonemic awareness and maturation of decoding skill, for instance, show reciprocity, as do, at a later point in reading development, levels of vocabulary knowledge and reading skill. We might now explore the relationship between two sides of written language: reading and writing: How do those processes correspond? Orthogonal to the relationship between reading and writing is the distinction between spoken language and written language. The written-language system shared by reading and writing is, as we have noted, an invented construct, as are its phonics and orthographic systems—and as are the conventions that readers and writers must learn in order to access and process written language. The spoken language, in contrast, is associated with a natural body of knowledge on which the written system is founded. Speakers and readers bring full and complete knowledge of spoken-language principles and of its systems (phonology, morphology, syntax, and semantics) to the spoken discourse context; that knowledge is implicit in speaking and listening behaviors, but it is not referenced explicitly. Knowledge of spoken-language principles and abstractions must become explicit, however, in order to be applied to written-language practices: to reading and writing.

Fitzgerald and Shanahan note the historical separation of those practices—of text production (writing) and text apprehension (reading)—in scholarship and in education, but they adduce the connectedness of the two fields in a shared knowledge base and shared processes (39). They adduce, too, reports of experimental interventions in which training on a task in one modality in a shared knowledge domain engenders growth in the other modality; for instance, sentence-combining training in writing tasks has been observed to improve reading comprehension of sentences (42). Building on Chall's model of reading development, Fitzgerald and Shanahan develop a functional model of written-language development that highlights the distinctive shared features at each stage and the recognition that those features—and the relation between reading and writing—modulate during development.

The first stage (birth through age six) of *literacy roots* corresponds to Chall's prereading stage. During this period of emergent literacy, children begin to amass implicit and explicit procedural and domain knowledge and, crucially, an early phonological and graphemic knowledge base on which reading and writing skills will be founded. The second stage (ages six to seven) of *initial literacy* corresponds to Chall's decoding stage, in which children learn letters and gain knowledge about letters and letter patterns; they begin to learn about the orthographic representation of spoken language's morphemic level. Crucial during this stage is the establishment of the phoneme–grapheme correspondence knowledge on which productive reading and writing depend. During this initial literacy stage, children progress through the series of spelling periods discussed in Chapter 2, moving from a semiphonetic spelling stance to phonetic and transitional spelling (cf. Moats 35–40). In the next written-language stage, under Fitzgerald and Shanahan's model, conventional (morphophonemic) spelling emerges; crucial in that third stage of *confirmation* (ages seven to eight), which corresponds to Chall's confirmation stage of reading, is the development of the procedural strategies underlying automaticity and fluency gains. Students learn to access and integrate process knowledge and learned strategies automatically, in order to achieve fluency in reading and writing.

As the confirmation stage progresses, moreover, the reader/writer, in preparation for a new type of procedural skill in the upcoming stage, is gaining more complex substantive knowledge, learning, for instance, the more advanced orthographic patterns that reflect the more complex morphology of "big words" (45). Knowledge of those "bigger ... academic, abstract words that appear in books" (46–47) is important to mastery of the procedural knowledge that is a focus in the fourth stage (ages nine to thirteen) of *reading and writing for learning the new.* At this stage, in which the roles of reading and writing in the apprehension and exposition of ideas are emphasized, self-monitoring procedures are important, as are knowledge of vocabulary, of complex syntactic forms that appear in written language, and of diverse text structures. Those acquisitions grow even more prominent in the fifth stage of *multiple viewpoints* (ages fourteen through eighteen): Procedural knowledge involving perspective shift, analytic/critical expression and interpretation, and revision strategies gain importance. And in the sixth stage (ages eighteen and above) of *construction and reconstruction,* content knowledge deepens; procedural knowledge growth permits the synthesis of ideas in the context of purposeful reading and writing.

Fitzgerald and Shanahan suggest that instruction capitalize on the connections between the two modalities at each stage of this developmental model of reading and writing; for instance, intervention targeting shared domain knowledge in one modality could be incorporated in practices that would support growth in both modalities (48). That enrichment potential is explored by Graham and Hebert, who analyze the impact of the "often-overlooked tool" (711) of writing by studying investigations of the effects of writing activities or writing instruction on reading skill development. In results that lend support to Fitzgerald and Shanahan's model of reading–writing connectedness, Graham and Hebert observe enhanced comprehension of reading materials that students have written about, improved reading outcomes in association with writing instruction, and the positive effect of overall quantity of assigned writing on reading comprehension levels during the elementary years.

The functional and developmental connectedness between reading and writing that is reflected in Fitzgerald and Shanahan's model of literacy growth is apparent, too, in literacy challenge. The dyslexic learner's struggle with literacy encompasses the full terrain of written language; the inhibiting effect of the core phonological processing deficit is indifferent to modality. Unable to perceive the speech stream as a phonemic sequence, the learner cannot make sense of the orthographic code that maps graphemes onto phonemes, and basic reading and spelling processes are rendered opaque. The review of treatment programs in Chapter 4 reveals, however, that clinicians, deeply aware that reading and writing share the impact of phonological processing challenge, are also attuned to the benefits of instruction that capitalizes on the reading–writing connection. Multimodal instruction is integral in Orton–Gillingham, LiPS, and RAVE-O programming. In the simultaneous oral spelling activity that represents a component of the Orton–Gillingham lesson, for example, phonemic segmentation is practiced on a spelling word: The learner sounds out the word while tapping for each phoneme. Proceeding to write the word's spelling while naming each letter, the learner is drawing a connection from phonemic segmentation to writing; reading the word back, the learner extends the connection to reading.

We see, too, that Fitzgerald and Shanahan's early stages mark a particularly sensitive period for the dyslexic learner. At the stage of literacy roots, the child should be building phonemic awareness and graphemic knowledge to support entry into reading and writing growth; at the initial literacy stage, the child should be developing the knowledge of phonics and orthographic conventions that will underlie advances in reading and writing. And the child in the confirmation stage will be acquiring, crucially, the strategic and integrative procedures that will permit growth in reading and writing automaticity and fluency. Reviewing the treatment programs, we note that the Lindamood LiPS program emphasizes the establishment of the phonological awareness and graphemic knowledge base for reading and writing that signals the literacy roots stage. The Orton–Gillingham program, while strengthening phoneme awareness, emphasizes the systematic development and activation of orthographic and phonics knowledge characterizing reading and writing growth during the initial literacy stage; the RAVE-O program, while sustaining training in phonemic awareness and phonics knowledge, emphasizes knowledge of the orthographic patterns and the orthographic reflexes of morphological structures that are consulted as automaticity and fluency in reading and writing develop during the confirmation stage.

The stages in Fitzgerald and Shanahan's model represent the growth stages through which the typical reader/writer passes when advancing to full literacy. The dyslexic reader/writer travels this route as well but is detained, as we have seen, by the struggle to achieve the insight of phonemic segmentation and to activate the phonemic awareness that will support phonics learning and application and, subsequently, the development of fluency in reading and writing that must precede reading and writing to learn the new.

Dyslexia and Writing

In their developmental model, Fitzgerald and Shanahan detail the complexity—the complexities—of the reading and writing of connected text. On the writing side, because the production of written text requires that the writer work on multiple levels, concerns at those various levels must often be addressed simultaneously. In the writing process, we can distinguish between higher-level composition skills—textual planning and organization, formulation of ideas, and coherence monitoring, for instance—and lower-level transcription skills—handwriting and spelling. Graham et al. point out the liabilities, during the elementary developmental years, that inhere in the multifaceted task of text production: The writer who has not yet mastered the mechanical skills involved in "getting language onto paper" (170) must dedicate attention to those mechanical processes, and this diversion of attention may strain working-memory processing capacity, such that higher-order composition performance is impacted (170). As Berninger et al. ("Writing Problems") note, the resources of working memory are limited, yet the demands of written composition are immense (8). At the early levels of writing growth, typically developing writers encounter this competition for working-memory space. Graham et al., studying children's composition fluency, found that young writers' composing fluency was affected directly by handwriting and spelling performance constraints in the early grades but that only handwriting performance had a significant effect on composition fluency in the intermediate grades. Composition quality in both the early and the middle years, moreover, was affected only by handwriting fluency (180).

The dyslexic writer, whose composition challenges are notorious (cf. Shaywitz), registers, likewise, the compromising effect of challenged transcription skills on composition output. Berninger et al. ("Writing Problems") recognize the challenge faced by dyslexic writers and underscore the significance of that challenge, observing, as does Shaywitz, those cases in which dyslexic students' reading challenge is mitigated, yet those students continue to struggle with spelling and composition. Berninger et al. note that although spelling difficulty is cited in the IDA definition of dyslexia, reading is often the focus in diagnosis and treatment. Dyslexia is conceptualized as a disorder of reading, but Berninger et al. adduce dyslexic children's below-mean performance on writing measures (3). In order to better understand that writing outcome by identifying the source(s) of performance deficit, they examined the relationship patterns among the various writing skills in dyslexic children and adults.

Berninger et al. ("Writing Problems") ground their research and their findings in the *simple view of writing* described by Berninger et al. ("Teaching Spelling" 292). This view is modeled as a triangle whose left-hand base vertex represents transcription skills (handwriting and spelling skills) and whose right-hand base vertex represents executive-function skills (self-regulation and planning skills); these lower-level skills support the higher-level text-generation skills represented at the upper vertex. Crucially, in this model of skill dynamic and skill integration across levels, the triangle's interior space represents working memory; fluent transcription skills permit limited working-memory resources to be allocated to composition: We see "transcription and self-regulation working together for the goal of text generation in working memory" (Berninger et al., "Teaching Spelling" 293). The triangle arms represent the connected relationships and transactions among the various writing components, in the context of the shared resources of limited working memory. Thus, for instance, automaticity in transcription skills permits the direction of working-memory resources toward the self-regulation strategies of planning, monitoring, and reviewing.

We saw that Graham et al., investigating interrelationships among typical children's handwriting, spelling, and composing performance, found that it was only handwriting automaticity—and not spelling—that made a crucial contribution to composition quality in typical beginning and developing writers in grades 1–6. Examining performance in dyslexic children and adults, Berninger et al. ("Writing Problems") looked at patterns in dyslexic writers' measured skills to determine whether the transcription skills of handwriting and spelling would relate in the same way to composition performance. Results on dyslexic writers, however, showed a different pattern. The children were all impaired in the handwriting, spelling, and written composition areas; the adults were less significantly impaired. In a finding that has substantial theoretical and clinical implications, spelling rather than handwriting was the unique predictor of the dyslexic writers' composition performance. And graphomotor planning, moreover, was also measured but made no unique contribution to composition performance: Graphomotor planning, which did make a unique contribution to typical children's composition results in earlier research, explained no additional variance in the outcome for dyslexic learners (Berninger et al., "Writing Problems" 11). The dyslexic learner's writing issues cannot be explained as a graphomotor challenge.

These results are important from both a research and a clinical perspective. From the point of view of science, they shed light on the etiology of a facet of dyslexic presentation that is well known to those who work in the field of dyslexia: Writing is an area of great vulnerability for the dyslexic individual. The learner who struggles with dyslexia encounters challenge not only in the apprehension of text but also in its production. And that difficulty occurs at the word level—in spelling—and at the textual level—in composing. In addition, however, the handwriting of a dyslexic learner is characteristically poor, and that impoverishment invites the inference that *dysgraphia*—specific handwriting challenge—is associated with dyslexic writing and with dyslexia. Berninger et al. ("Writing Problems") state that the children in the study showed handwriting as well as spelling impairment; crucially, however, it was spelling rather than handwriting that accounted for variation in composition performance. As we have seen, "disastrous spelling" is a hallmark of dyslexia—as is "messy handwriting." Often accompanying that sloppy handwriting, however, are "nimble fingers" (Shaywitz 124). It has been well established that the spelling challenge in dyslexia has its source in the core phonological processing deficit; the concomitant sloppy handwriting and agile fingers, however—and the absence of a direct connection between graphomotor planning and composition performance in Berninger et al.'s results—suggest that the reduced quality of dyslexic handwriting presentation is not due to dysgraphia. Dysgraphia, or persistent handwriting impairment, is, like dyslexia, a learning difference; it is signaled by impaired letter-form production, leading to illegible handwriting and labored writing. Those writing difficulties associated with dysgraphia may result in spelling or composition challenge but are not accompanied by reading challenge.

A vital research insight in Berninger et al.'s ("Writing Problems") finding that spelling issues rather than handwriting issues explained unique variance in dyslexic writing outcomes is that it is spelling rather than handwriting difficulty that underlies the broader writing vulnerability in dyslexia. Spelling challenge affects handwriting: Challenged spellers hesitate during writing, and letter production becomes less fluent. And spelling challenge affects composition quality by, for instance, reducing lexical diversity in the written product. Berninger et al. ("Writing Problems") note the constraining effect, in conceptual exposition, of spelling challenge when writers restrict their lexical selection to "the words they think they can spell without embarrassment" (13). This insight in turn informs clinical practice; in the case of writing challenge, accurate diagnosis that will differentiate between the dyslexic and the dysgraphic writer is imperative. For the dyslexic writer, treatment must address both spelling and the compromised phonological processing skill that is limiting spelling growth.

Richards et al. arrive at results that support further the conclusion that the dyslexic writer and the dysgraphic writer, both challenged writers, are associated with distinct profiles; accurate diagnosis must differentiate the two learners in order to ensure appropriate treatment. To confirm the clinical differentiation, Richards et al. compared neurological profiles (409). They studied a group of children in grades 4–9 who had been diagnosed with dysgraphia, another group of children diagnosed with dyslexia, and a control group of children whose writing and reading skills were typical. Clinically, children in both the dysgraphic group and the dyslexic group were challenged in spelling. Spelling challenge accompanied vitiated decoding in the dyslexic group; the spelling skill reduction accompanied impaired handwriting in the dysgraphic group, but the dysgraphic learners had no decoding issues. Richards et al. administered handwriting, spelling, and cognitive tasks; the children wrote with a fiber-optic pen so that researchers could maintain a real-time record of their writing. At the same time, brain activity was measured through functional magnetic resonance imaging (fMRI); neurological profiles were examined during the handwriting and spelling tasks for comparisons on "white matter integrity, functional connectivity, and white matter–gray matter correlations" (Richards et al. 409).

Results, again, were important from both a research and a clinical perspective: The neurological finding, which "adds to the rapidly expanding knowledge of the heavily connected brain ... by showing that structural connections and functional connections are related in differential and complex ways in children with and without dysgraphia and dyslexia" (Richards et al. 420), was that while completing the written-language and cognitive tasks, the typical children in the control group displayed a greater number of the white-matter cerebral connections that scaffold gray-matter functional connections dedicated to language and cognitive processes. The children in both the dyslexia and the dysgraphia groups, on the other hand, displayed fewer white-matter connections and a greater number of functional connections to gray-matter sites, revealing less efficient task response: They invested greater neural effort to complete the written-language and cognitive tasks. Equally important, the children in the dyslexia and dysgraphia groups also differed by group during both the writing and the cognitive task performances, contrasting in white-matter connections and patterns, and in the gray-matter functional connection levels. These results indicate that dysgraphia and dyslexia represent distinct impairments: Both are associated with handwriting impairment, but that shared deficit appears in the context of different clinical presentations, reflected in neurological difference.

We can understand the divergent dysgraphic and dyslexic clinical presentations in terms of the model of the simple view of writing (Berninger et al., "Teaching Spelling" 292): Writers in both groups are challenged by the transcription skills of handwriting and spelling, yet those double challenges have different sources. The primary challenge of the dysgraphic writer is handwriting, and that impairment exhausts the limited working-memory resources that cannot then be applied to spelling. The converse holds in the case of the dyslexic writer, whose primary challenge is spelling; hesitant spelling slows handwriting and also appropriates working-memory resources that might have been invested in handwriting. Accompanying—and underlying—these divergent clinical profiles, moreover, are structural and functional neural differences. This result argues for accurate and differentiated diagnosis that in turn calls for differentiated and individualized treatment plans:

> Neuroscience research has an important societal contribution to make in educating educators and policy makers that these brain-based SLDs [specific learning disabilities] affecting writing—dysgraphia and dyslexia—exist, can be diagnosed, have different brain bases ... and deserve individually tailored instruction.
>
> (Richards et al. 420)

The learner ages in this study, moreover, indicate that handwriting and spelling problems persist; that persistence directs educators toward systematic treatment plans and the individualized, explicit methods that have been so successful in therapeutic programming.

Amplifying our understanding of the dyslexic writer, the research findings reported by Berninger et al. ("Writing Problems") and Richards et al. sharpen our focus on spelling. The dyslexic writer, challenged by higher-level composing skills and lower-level transcription skills, struggles at all levels of the complex project that writing represents, yet we see that spelling performance often explains performance in other areas, accounting directly, for instance, for variance in composing success. Given the persistence of spelling issues in dyslexia, such results suggest a close look at spelling: at its relation to reading, at the spelling profile of the dyslexic learner, and at the ways in which spelling performance interfaces with other writing outcomes.

Reading and Spelling

Fitzgerald and Shanahan call attention to the functional and developmental connections between reading and writing. As we narrow our focus to spelling, we see that Ehri brings into focus the relatedness of reading and spelling, observing that "learning to read and learning to spell are one and same, almost" (237). She remarks on the many faces of spelling: *Spelling* signifies not only an activity but also an orthographic sequence that is both the product of spelling and the object of reading, and the spelling task itself can represent an expressive behavior (retrieving the letter sequence) or a recognition behavior (determining whether a given sequence is an accurate orthographic rendition of a word) (238). Expressive spelling, for the skilled speller, is often followed by self-monitoring in which the speller reads back the orthographic sequence to confirm its accuracy—"to see whether it 'looks right'" (Perfetti 24). In the expressive spelling task, we are asked to spell; in spelling recognition, we read. These points of contact suggest that reading and spelling are closely connected: We read spellings, we spell spellings, and we read back spellings to assess them for conformity with convention (Ehri 238).

Ehri examines the ways in which skilled readers and spellers process words: For either spelling or reading purposes, words are processed "by memory, by invention, [or] by analogy" (240). Familiar words are spelled or read by *memory*, in an automatic response to a word whose representation is stored as a single unit in lexical memory. *Invention* involves decoding in the case of reading and encoding in the case of spelling: Applying the sound–symbol code, the pronunciation of an unfamiliar word is assembled from the sequenced sounds associated with its letters; the orthography of an unfamiliar word is constructed from the letter sequence associated with its sounds. An unfamiliar word can also be read or spelled by means of *analogy* with a familiar word; Moats points out that the maturing speller increasingly favors the analogy strategy (45). This observation underscores the importance, in skilled spelling, of reading experience and vocabulary development: Both enrich the supply of word units stored in the speller's lexical memory; the orthographic patterns are available for analogical comparison.

The different processing strategies are associated not only with diverse application contexts (familiar and unfamiliar words) but also with diverse types of knowledge. Spelling by analogy depends on a rich store of remembered and accessible lexical forms; systemic knowledge—knowledge of sound–symbol relationships and of orthographic patterns—is crucial to the invention approach. Under the memory approach, the speller also consults the word-specific knowledge stored in word representations in lexical memory. Ehri points out, however, that word-specific knowledge, although resulting from reading and spelling encounters with words, is also dependent on alphabetic knowledge—on knowledge of the spelling system: "Knowledge of the system functions as a mnemonic tool, enabling students to retain letter-specific information about individual words in memory" (244). Under

Ehri's approach, the lexical representations, although single word units, are alphabetic representations in which graphemes are bonded to phonemes. The bonded grapheme–phoneme connection permits accurate and automatic retrieval of a single pronunciation response for reading, yet spelling and reading diverge here. When the speller responds to a pronunciation by accessing the lexical representation of the word for spelling, the spelling response is multiple rather than singular: The speller retrieves multiple, sequenced individual letters for the spelling (247). If the speller omits letters, the spelling is inaccurate; accurate reading will be easier than accurate spelling.

We see, under Ehri's model of reading and spelling, strategy-specific activation of different processes and of diverse types of knowledge as the reader and the speller consult both word-specific information and general conventions of the grapheme–phoneme correspondence system. Because the word-specific listings are orthographic representations in which graphemes are bonded to phonemes, both types of knowledge rely on phonics application and alphabetic word representations, highlighting the code-based and code-reliant foundation of reading and spelling. Ehri also reports reading–spelling and spelling–reading transactions (257–261). She observes that reading affects spelling in young learners: Reading provides the opportunity for learners to acquire the word-specific knowledge applied in spelling tasks. In young learners, likewise, spelling practice supports reading growth; Ehri hypothesizes that this is so because spelling practice strengthens (alphabetic) systemic knowledge. Because word-specific knowledge is, under Ehri's model, coded alphabetically, the learning transfer in both directions attests to the mediating role of code knowledge. In skilled learners, spelling and reading share a strong and reciprocal relationship; accurate spelling is just a little harder than reading because it draws more heavily on memory: "Failure," Ehri states, "to remember one or two letters dooms a perfect spelling but not necessarily an accurate reading" (248). If a phoneme in a lexical item is associated with more than one graphemic reflex, the conventionally designated grapheme will be harder to store and retrieve and thus will more likely challenge memory in a spelling task; silent and doubled letters in a lexical string and uncommon orthographic patterns, likewise, will vitiate spelling fluency (248).

Pursuing further the perspective that reading and spelling are "two sides of a coin" (28), Perfetti models the relationship between reading and spelling; the two behaviors have the same lexicon base and diverge in their processing. Both depend on high-quality orthographic representations associated with individual listings in the lexicon; the quality of those representations resides in the *"precision* and *redundancy"* in lexical listings. Precision involves the completeness and accuracy of the letter-sequence representation of a word in the lexicon, Ehri's word-specific information; redundancy appears in the grapheme–phoneme associations that are, under Ehri's analysis, bonded connections stored in lexical memory. The reiteration in two types of orthography–phonology connections—between printed and spoken units at the word level, and between the word-specific graphemic and phonemic segments at the phonemic level—ensures reading and spelling success and fluency. As Perfetti points out, both precision and redundancy are strengthened through literacy experience. And the establishment of representations that feature precision and redundancy requires phonological knowledge: awareness at the phonemic level.

In Perfetti's model, as in Ehri's account, spelling will be more difficult than reading. Recognizing the significance of the mapping difference, such that the phonology–orthography mapping consulted in spelling is more diverse than is the orthography–phonology mapping activated in reading, and of the more stringent accuracy requirement in spelling, such that reading can be successful even in the case of an incomplete lexical representation, Perfetti acknowledges the singular challenge of the grapheme retrieval process; spelling calls for grapheme retrieval rather than the grapheme recognition called on in reading (30). On the other hand, the two processes utilize the same lexical representation; in addition, Perfetti argues, both spelling and reading incorporate verification strategies. The accuracy of a produced spelling is verified via readback; Perfetti also adduces the case of reading verification via spelling (34). In Chapter 1, the cross-modal effect of orthography on spoken-word processing, recorded by Ziegler and Ferrand, and later by Ziegler et al., was observed in the effect of alternative spelling options for a phonological segment on listener response time. Perfetti points to another instance in which the presence of orthographic alternatives affects response time—as a within-modality *feedback* effect, in this case. In models of word identification, a *feedforward* effect has been observed: Words containing graphemic segments whose mapping to phonemic segments is ambiguous—words with letters/letter clusters that could be pronounced in more than one way—are read more slowly, suggesting that skilled readers continue to consult sound–symbol mappings during the reading process. Stone et al. also observe a *feedback* effect: In a lexical-decision task, subjects who were asked to read a displayed printed word responded more slowly on words with orthographic alternatives—words that might have been spelled in another way. This observed feedback effect suggests that a reading is accompanied by spelling verification—a spelling feedback step in which the phonology–orthography match is checked—that will proceed less efficiently if the presented spelling has viable competitors.

In the context of a broader reading–writing connectedness, the relatedness of spelling to reading is apparent in typical development: in literacy functions, in shared growth stages, and in a shared reference to grapheme–phoneme correspondences that is pertinent throughout development and at skilled levels. The speller shares with the reader an early dependence on the achievement of the phonemic insight and activation of the phonemic awareness that will permit phonics learning and its application to literacy tasks. Spelling and reading processes consult a single set of listings stored in lexical memory and the same types of knowledge: word-specific knowledge and conventional knowledge of the grapheme–phoneme correspondence system. Lexically stored orthographic forms that are accessed for spelling and for reading have precision and redundancy features that add quality to the representations, and the stored listings accrue with amassed reading and spelling experiences. Crucially, reading and spelling are—persistently—code-reliant and code-based processes. And spelling, in models of typical development, will be harder than reading. The connectedness of reading and spelling and the increment of challenge in spelling's grapheme retrieval requirement explain the vulnerable status of spelling skill in dyslexia, such that spelling issues are cited in the IDA definition of dyslexia, such that they persist in the written-language profile of a student like Hayden, and such that spelling is often the ultimate challenge for the dyslexic learner and, often, the last skill to respond to treatment (cf., e.g., Shaywitz 114).

Dyslexia and Spelling

Reading and spelling are deeply connected functionally, neurologically, and clinically. Reliant on phonological processing competence, both represent areas of vulnerability for the dyslexic learner; for both typical and dyslexic learners, spelling often represents the greater challenge. We have seen, too, that spelling plays a special role for the dyslexic learner in writing achievement. Of the transcription skills of handwriting and spelling, handwriting was found by Graham et al. to be the only contributor to composition quality in the output of typical primary- and intermediate-grade writers. Berninger et al. ("Writing Problems") observed a different skill pattern in dyslexic writers, however: It was spelling rather than handwriting that accounted for unique variance in the dyslexic writers' composition performance. Dyslexic writers evince challenge in handwriting and composition as well as in spelling (Shaywitz 254), yet Berninger et al. found spelling challenge to be the preeminent source of reduction in the writing product. Under the assumptions of the simple view of writing (Berninger et al., "Teaching Spelling" 292) regarding the competition for limited working-memory resources during writing, the excessive demands of spelling on the dyslexic writer divert those resources so that they are unavailable for other tasks and at other levels in the writing processes.

How does the dyslexic speller spell? In earlier discussion of the written-language profile (Chapter 3), the contrast between dysphonetic and dyseidetic misspellings was adduced. A dysphonetic spelling is phonetically implausible; it represents an orthographic string that is inconsistent with the target word's phonological sequence. A dyseidetic spelling, in contrast, is consistent with the phonological sequence in a lexical item but ignores the conventional orthography. Like the routes to misspelling, the avenues to spelling achievement are diverse: A speller may be guided by sound and/or by letter patterns. In an alphabetic orthography like that of English, phonological sequence informs orthography; phonologic–orthographic pairings are mediated by phonics knowledge of systematic phoneme–grapheme associations. Access to the phonemic level of language is thus crucial to spelling success.

English, however, multiplex in its history and expansive in its lexicon, has a deep orthography; phonemic–graphemic coding is necessary but not sufficient for accurate conventional spelling. The phoneme–grapheme code itself is complicated in that a single grapheme may be associated with multiple pronunciations (e.g., the grapheme *c* can be realized as the phonemes /s/ or /k/), and a single phoneme may yield multiple graphemic reflexes (e.g., the phoneme /k/ may be represented as *c, k, ch*, or *q*). Word-specific conventions may assign an orthographic sequence to a word whose encoding is not fully determined via application of sound–symbol phonics conventions, yet orthographic coding appears at levels other than the phonemic level. English spelling, as we have seen, is morphophonemic: Both phonemes and morphemes are referenced in orthographic coding. Orthographic coding of morphology involves systematic encoding of certain morphemes; the past-tense inflectional suffix, for example, is coded as the orthographic unit *–ed* rather than being coded phonetically as *d* or *t* or *id*. Other units of natural language may be recognized orthographically; for instance, the word-final syllable in words like *table* or *trifle* is encoded as the orthographic unit *consonant-le*. In addition to memory for word-specific spellings, awareness of morphological coding conventions, and sensitivity to syllabic structures, moreover, knowledge of *graphotactic* regularities—licensed letter patterns—contributes to successful spelling. Graphotactic knowledge is knowledge of letter-distribution generalities: awareness of letter sequences permitted by orthographic convention. Characteristically, for instance, English words do not begin with doubled consonants and do not end in *j*.

Given dyslexic learners' vitiated access to a phonemic representation of the speech stream and, therefore, to fluent application of phonics generalizations when spelling, we might expect that dyslexic spellers would rely more heavily on orthographic strategies. Researchers have pursued this idea, matching groups of dyslexic spellers and groups of typical (younger) spellers by spelling age in order to examine the interaction of spelling behavior and phonological processing capacity in the dyslexic spelling group. Asking whether dyslexic spellers and typical spellers differ not only in their access to phonemic knowledge but also in spelling strategy, Cassar et al. tested the hypothesis that dyslexic spellers rely more heavily than do typical spellers on graphotactic knowledge, arriving at spellings that "'look right' even when they do not represent the sounds of the target words" (28). Those spellers, matched with typical spellers on real-word spelling performance, would be less successful on measures invoking phonological processing—on phonemic awareness tests and on the spelling of orthographically transparent nonwords—but more successful on measures of graphotactic knowledge. Phonological processing skill was measured in a phoneme-counting task and a nonword-spelling task involving repeating and then writing the spelling for an orally presented nonword. Graphotactic knowledge was measured in a spelling-choice test in which children circled the word in a pair of four-letter nonwords that "looked more like real words should look" (33). The targeted graphotactic knowledge about English involved various letter sequences that either were allowed (e.g., word-initial *dr* or the doublet *ss*) or did not appear in English (e.g., word-initial *gv* or the doublet *vv*).

Cassar et al.'s findings shed light on the skill profiles of the dyslexic spellers, relative to the profiles of typical, younger spellers with whom they were matched by real-word spelling achievement. Misspelling analyses in the two groups revealed that the parity observed in overall real-word spelling achievement appeared as well in characteristic misspellings on particular challenges such as the spellings for reduced vowels (unstressed vowels with a neutral pronunciation and diverse graphemic reflexes, such as the *e* in *dozen* or the *i* in *pencil*) or the spelled representations (e.g., *bl-* or *-nd*) of consonant sound clusters. Parity extended, too, to performance on phonological processing measures such as the nonword-spelling and phoneme-counting tasks. Likewise, moreover, the two groups did not differ in graphotactic knowledge level, as displayed in the spelling-choice task and in the degree to which permitted letter sequences characterized expressive spelling responses. To confirm these findings, Cassar et al. utilized another measure: teacher judgment. Asking experienced teachers to judge, on the basis of spelling responses on the real-word spelling measures, whether the speller was a younger typical student or an older dyslexic student, Cassar et al. found that teachers could not distinguish typical beginning spellers from older dyslexic spellers on the basis of the children's spellings. This result corroborates the finding that the spelling performances in the two groups were similar: There was no evidence of spelling strategies, strengths, and/or challenges that distinguished the spelling outputs of the two groups.

Cassar et al.'s results indicate that dyslexic spellers perform at a reduced level for age but struggle with the same spelling issues that challenge typical early spellers. Their phonological processing skills, moreover, were on a par with those of the typical younger spellers, suggesting a match not only in spelling achievement but also in phonological processing capability. This result in turn underscores the intimate connection between phonological processing skill and spelling achievement, such that "knowledge about the spelling patterns of a language is laid over a phonological foundation" (43). These findings suggest the consequences of the Matthew effect (Stanovich), applied to spelling achievement:

> Because of their poor phonological skills, children with dyslexia do not readily grasp the basis of an alphabetic writing system and do not acquire a sizable store of written spellings. This, in turn, means that they do not have a good database from which to learn about the letter patterns of the language.
>
> (Cassar et al. 45)

The gap between dyslexic spellers and their typical age peers will only grow as the dyslexic students' spelling experience and spelling growth languish.

The clinical ramifications are evident: The prospect of an accelerating spelling-achievement deficit argues for treatment that addresses spelling skills in dyslexic writers and that is also directed toward the concomitant phonological processing deficit. In addition, though, Cassar et al. observe that the similarity between the challenges that dyslexic spellers encounter and the areas of difficulty for typical early spellers suggests that spelling treatment for dyslexic spellers need not differ in character from the instruction offered to typical spellers (46). That treatment would, however, be distinguished by its concentration and persistence: Code-based spelling instruction for the dyslexic speller must be focused, explicit, and systematic; addressing phonological processing skill directly, it must also address those areas of challenge that all spellers encounter.

The findings of Cassar et al., like those of Berninger et al. ("Writing Problems"), call attention to the primacy of spelling issues in the written-language profile of the dyslexic learner and underscore the importance of phonological processing skill development, foundational to spelling growth. Spelling achievement is not only a key index in the diagnosis of dyslexia but also a foundational transcription skill that impacts written composition performance: Berninger et al. show that spelling challenge in the dyslexic writer predicts written composition performance. Sumner et al. ("The Influence of Spelling Ability"), like Berninger et al., direct attention to the predictive role of spelling in composition outcomes, investigating more closely the association between spelling achievement and written composition performance and revealing that the connection between spelling and composition is mediated by performance in other aspects of writing. In earlier work ("Children with Dyslexia"), Sumner et al. found that dyslexic children not only made more spelling errors during narrative composition but also paused more frequently while spelling than did typical age-peer writers, such that handwriting was slowed by spelling pauses. Hesitant spelling, slowing handwriting, reduced composing fluency and quality. Handwriting thus mediates the association between spelling level and composition performance.

Another aspect of writing that contributes to composition quality but is sensitive to spelling challenge is vocabulary: The lexical diversity in vocabulary selection enriches a composition. In earlier discussion, we noted Berninger et al.'s comment that when composing, challenged spellers constrain lexical choices to "the words they think they can spell without embarrassment" ("Writing Problems" 13), thereby limiting overall composition quality. Comparing a group of dyslexic writers to a spelling-age-matched group of writers and a chronological-age-matched writer group, Sumner et al. ("The Influence of Spelling Ability") postulated, following the simple view of writing (Berninger et al., "Teaching Spelling"), that challenges in the lower-level transcription processes of handwriting and spelling drain working-memory resources during written composition; they explored this additional way in which spelling challenge might affect lexical diversity in the writing product. The writers utilized a digital writing tablet so that writer pauses during composition, which would register spelling difficulty, could be tracked. Children in the three study groups were asked to compose both a written and an oral composition.

The dyslexic students resembled the spelling-matched students on certain measures: They were on a par with the younger writers in spelling error count but made significantly more errors than did the age-matched writers. As in earlier work ("Children with Dyslexia"), Sumner et al. ("The Influence of Spelling Ability") observed pauses when the dyslexic children wrote, finding a correlation between spelling skill reduction and pauses while writing. In the written compositions, the dyslexic writers' vocabulary was more constrained than that of the age-matched writers, although vocabulary was even more restricted in the written compositions of the younger, spelling-matched writers. The dyslexic writers' lexical diversity on the written task increased, moreover, with spelling achievement. In the dyslexic group, spelling level and pauses explained 53 percent of the variance in lexical diversity, indicating that the reduced lexical diversity was a consequence of spelling challenge, although spelling skill did not predict lexical diversity in either the age- or the spelling-matched control groups. Of interest were the quality ratings on both the written and the oral compositions. On the written compositions, children in the dyslexic group were rated on a par with younger spelling-matched writers and at a lower level than the age-matched writers. Quality ratings for the dyslexic writers and for their spelling peers were stronger on the oral compositions; in their oral compositions, dyslexic students showed an age-appropriate vocabulary level, although vocabulary was more impoverished in their written work. Their age peers, however, were rated more highly on their written work than on their oral compositions.

These results reveal the toll that spelling vulnerability exacts. Associations among lexical diversity level, spelling performance, and pause rate indicated that the dyslexic writers' lexical diversity on the written composition was contingent on spelling ability. Elevated within-word pause rate registered spelling difficulty; the more impoverished lexical diversity that accompanied elevation in spelling error count and pause rate suggests that limited working-memory resources were being expended on spelling during the transcription process and were not available for vocabulary selection. The higher quality ratings on the dyslexic students' oral compositions were not significantly different from those on their age peers' oral compositions, suggesting a modality effect: For the dyslexic writers, the written mode—and the drain on attention resources due to spelling challenge—reduced access to vocabulary options that were available during the oral composition process.

Cassar et al.'s findings, recognizing the familiar challenge of single-word spelling for the dyslexic writer, shed light on that challenge: Like the typical speller, the dyslexic speller must access the phonemic level of language in order to apply the sound–symbol regularities underlying alphabetic spelling.

Phonological processing limitations make spelling more difficult, yet the dyslexic speller encounters the same spelling issues that confront the typical speller. When the dyslexic writer engages in the multilevel composition process, however, the impact of spelling challenge is magnified. Because spelling difficulty affects handwriting fluency and vocabulary selection, composition quality and fluency are compromised. Summer et al. ("Children with Dyslexia") observe the mediating effect on handwriting performance: Dysfluent spelling constrains speed in handwriting, thereby reducing composing fluency and quality. Vocabulary, too, may mediate the effect of spelling challenge on composing: Berninger et al. ("Writing Problems") remark that dyslexic writers limit their lexical selection to those words they can spell confidently. In addition, Summer et al. ("The Influence of Spelling Ability") show that the demands of spelling deplete working-memory reserves, diverting attention that might have been allocated to vocabulary selection; textual enrichment through lexical diversity is thereby sacrificed.

Writing Treatment

Because speech is easy, reading is hard; spelling is even harder. For the dyslexic reader-speller, spelling is especially—and persistently—difficult. Phonological processing at the phonemic level, fundamental at the entry into reading and writing, represents an area of vulnerability for that learner. The recognition of a grapheme string for reading, which is utilized during the spelling process for readback monitoring (cf. Perfetti 24), is associated with its own challenges, but the fully accurate retrieval of graphemes for spelling adds an increment of difficulty. And because spelling represents the first step toward writing and remains a foundational transcription skill that is exercised throughout the writing process, spelling skill affects written composition success at all levels. Throughout the writing process, the dyslexic writer is slowed by dysfluent spelling, yet so much energy is expended on that transcription skill that working memory resources are exhausted; attention cannot be directed toward the higher-level composing processes.

   The mechanisms by which the effects of spelling challenge radiate to other processes and other levels during the writing process can be understood in the framework of the simple view of writing. That model of the writing process, which incorporates the various writing skill areas—transcription, executive function, and composition—as vertices of a triangle enclosing a shared working-memory space, also represents the transactional relations among the skill areas as triangle arms. Berninger et al.'s ("Writing Problems") finding that for dyslexic writers, spelling was a unique predictor of composition performance can be understood as the outcome of a dynamic under which the dyslexic writer's hesitant spelling constrains automaticity in the other transcription skill of handwriting; at the same time, limited working-memory resources, expended on spelling, cannot be dedicated either to executive-function management of the writing process or to the

concerns of text generation and composition quality. Richards et al.'s identification of neurological profiles that distinguished dysgraphic and dyslexic
students can be understood as a case in which two types of writers share
challenge in the transcription skills of handwriting and spelling, yet that
ostensible similarity obscures a crucial difference: The fundamental handwriting impairment of the dysgraphic writer exhausts precious working-
memory resources that cannot then be expended on spelling; the fundamental spelling impairment of the dyslexic writer appropriates attentional
resources that cannot then be dedicated to handwriting.

Differential diagnosis, justified not only by differing constellations of
associated skills but also by distinct neurological profiles, is critical to the
design of appropriate treatment that must target the handwriting challenge
of the dysgraphic writer and the spelling challenge of the dyslexic writer.
The transcription issues present similarly but, distinguished clinically and
neurally, have divergent etiologies and require different therapies. Sumner et
al. ("Children with Dyslexia") observed that slowness in the transcription
skill of handwriting, attributable to a deficit in the other transcription skill
of spelling, impacts composition fluency; likewise, Sumner et al. ("The
Influence of Spelling Ability") found that composition quality, reduced by
restricted vocabulary, can be explained, ultimately, by that same transcription skill deficit: a spelling deficit.

Under the simple view of writing, the triangle vertices represent sites at
which challenge might occur; Berninger et al. also point out that the skill
areas of transcription, self-regulation, and text-generation suggest targets for
writing instruction ("Teaching Spelling," 293). In addition, remediation that
focuses on a challenge situated at one vertex can, by virtue of the connections between skill areas, ameliorate skills at another site. Spelling remediation in a dyslexic writer, for instance, might reduce pauses and thereby
ameliorate another transcription performance (handwriting), might free
working-memory resources for executive-function concerns such as planning
or reviewing, or might free resources for composition enrichment through
improved lexical diversity. The model, accommodating research findings,
also guides treatment design.

Hebert et al. ("Why Children with Dyslexia Struggle"), referencing the
connectedness of reading and writing and the shared processes underlying
both, note that the challenge that the dyslexic learner encounters in writing
is not unexpected. Reading, an area of vulnerability for that learner, is
called on not only in spelling verification but also at other points during the
writing process. The writer may need to read print sources for the writing
project; reading is required, too, during the review and revision processes.
Hebert et al. cite the dyslexic learner's writing concerns—"poor spelling,
poor legibility, lack of diverse vocabulary, poor idea development, and/or
lack of organization" (843)—and consider these writing issues in the context
of the simple view of writing, observing that the model provides a framework not only for an account of the multicomponential writing process but

also for treatment design (861). They consider both remediation and compensation: Remediation addresses a writing skill directly, reducing its deficit; compensation offers strategies whereby the demands of writing are reduced and the writing process is made more manageable (861). In the transcription skill area, for instance, discrete remediation treatments would address spelling and handwriting, whereas compensatory strategies might include keyboarding instruction.

The research findings of Berninger et al. ("Writing Problems"), Richards et al., and Sumner et al. ("The Influence of Spelling Ability") are instructive here: Accurate diagnosis is paramount. Accurate dysgraphia and dyslexia diagnoses, for instance, permit appropriate treatments in the two cases: handwriting remediation for the dysgraphic student and spelling remediation for the dyslexic student. Although both learners may display dysfluent handwriting, spelling impairment is the source of the dyslexic student's impairment, whereas handwriting challenge explains that of the dysgraphic student. Sumner et al. ("A Review of Dyslexia") emphasize that although the dyslexic child composes text more slowly than do peers, the handwriting speed itself is not reduced; instead, pauses slow the writing process. Spelling impairment has imposed restrictions on handwriting speed, and spelling remediation is called for. Spelling remediation would be appropriate, too, when a composition's quality is reduced due to impoverished lexical diversity, given the findings in Sumner et al. ("The Influence of Spelling Ability"). Selection of a key target for therapy, however, does not preclude additional instruction in an area where skill development has been compromised due to a deficit elsewhere; thus spelling remediation might be accompanied by vocabulary enrichment to enhance lexical diversity.

Executive-function issues during the writing process, such as challenges in the presentation or organization of ideas at the sentence or text level, might, like slow handwriting or absence of lexical diversity, be attributable to a drain on working-memory resources due to the demands of spelling issues. Spelling remediation would be vital; structural/organizational executive-function issues, however, might also be addressed directly. To remedy issues of organization and structure at the sentential level, Hebert et al. ("Why Children with Dyslexia Struggle") propose sentence-combining activities. In sentence combining, the student is given two or more simple sentences and is asked to combine them into a single (compound or complex) sentence that preserves the ideas in the simple structures. This strategy is an effective instructional tool that has been used to build textual planning and organizing skills at a range of educational levels; as a resource, Hebert et al. recommend *Teacher's Guide to Effective Sentence Planning*, by Bruce Saddler. They also suggest, as another executive-function support, *self-regulated strategy development* (SRSD); under SRSD, the student learns to utilize self-regulation, goal setting, self-speech, and self-monitoring in order to define, plan for, and execute a writing task (Hebert et al., "Why Children with Dyslexia Struggle" 857–858). An additional executive-function support is the

Structures Writing program for expository writing (cf., e.g., Hebert et al., "Writing Informational Text"). In order to reduce working-memory demands under this program, students are provided with content ideas and vocabulary while they are trained in text structures. The Structures Writing program also limits text organization choices to five options—description, compare/contrast, sequence, cause/effect, and problem/solution—so that the writer can dedicate working-memory resources to writing.

Writing and the Dyslexic Learner

Careful research and partnerships among scholars, clinicians, and educators have been crucial to the advances resulting in the current understanding of dyslexia, of its assessment, and of its treatment. The language user's full, complete, and implicit knowledge of natural language structures must become explicit in order for that learner to apprehend and apply the alphabetic conventions of English orthography; access to the phonemic structure of spoken language is foundational to mastery of the written conventions of reading and spelling. The core phonological processing deficit observed in dyslexia challenges achievement of the phonemic insight; the dyslexic learner therefore struggles to read and struggles even more to spell.

Studies of the dyslexic writer offer insight into the source of that writer's struggle when composing connected text: The problem of spelling, persistent at the single-word level, is amplified in the context of extended composition, consuming resources that might have been dedicated to the creation of content. The simple model of writing clarifies the role of spelling in the writing process and illuminates its disruptive potential. Equally powerful, however, are treatment options. The complex and multilevel project that writing represents adds complexity to diagnosis, and accurate diagnosis is critical—yet, when achieved, prefigures remediation. Because reading and spelling are deeply connected, the explicit, highly structured, code-based approaches like Orton–Gillingham, Lindamood–Bell LiPS, and RAVE-O that address spelling, reading, and the phonemic awareness that must serve literacy will work directly to retrain the dyslexic writer. Spelling is hard, profoundly hard for the dyslexic writer, but—as an element of the second-order written-language system—profoundly conventional. As an invented and conventional system, it is both teachable and learnable.

Works Cited

Berninger, Virginia W., Katherine Vaughan, Robert D. Abbott, Kristin Begay, Kristina Byrd Coleman, Gerald Curtin, Jill Minich Hawkins, and Steve Graham. "Teaching Spelling and Composition Alone and Together: Implications for the Simple View of Writing." *Journal of Educational Psychology* 94:2 (2002): 291–304.

Berninger, Virginia W., Kathleen H. Nielsen, Robert D. Abbott, Ellen Wijsman, and Ellen Raskind. "Writing Problems in Dyslexia: Under-Recognized and Under-Treated." *Journal of School Psychology* 46:1 (February 2008): 1–21.

Cassar, Marie, Rebecca Treiman, Louisa Moats, Tatiana Cury Pollo, and Brett Kessler. "How Do the Spellings of Children with Dyslexia Compare with Those of Nondyslexic Children?" *Reading and Writing* 18 (2005): 27–49.

Chall, Jeanne. *Stages of Reading Development*. New York: McGraw-Hill, 1983.

Ehri, Linnea. "Learning to Read and Learning to Spell Are One and the Same, Almost." *Learning to Spell: Research, Theory, and Practice Across Languages*. Eds. Charles A. Perfetti, Laurence Rieben, and Michel Foyol. Mahwah, NJ: Lawrence Erlbaum Associates, 1997. 237–269.

Fitzgerald, Jill, and Timothy Shanahan. "Reading and Writing Relations and Their Development." *Educational Psychologist* 35:1 (2000): 39–50.

Graham, Steve, Virginia W. Berninger, Robert D. Abbott, Sylvia P. Abbott, and Dianne Whitaker. "Role of Mechanics in Composing of Elementary School Students: A New Methodological Approach." *Journal of Educational Psychology* 89:1 (1997): 170–182.

Graham, Steve, and Michael Hebert. "Writing to Read: A Meta-Analysis of the Impact of Writing and Writing Instruction on Reading." *Harvard Educational Review* 81:4 (Winter 2011): 710–744.

Hebert, Michael, Janet J. Bohaty, Ron Nelson, and Julia V. Rohling. "Writing Informational Text Using Provided Information and Text Structures: An Intervention for Upper Elementary Struggling Writers." *Reading and Writing* 31:3 (April 2018): 2165–2190.

Hebert, Michael, Devin M. Kearns, Joanne Baker Hayes, Pamela Bazis, and Samantha Cooper. "Why Children with Dyslexia Struggle with Writing and How to Help Them." *Language, Speech, and Hearing Services in Schools* 48 (October 2018): 843–863.

Moats, Louisa Cooke. *Spelling: Development, Disability, and Instruction*. Timonium, MD: York Press, 1995.

Perfetti, Charles A. "The Psycholinguistics of Spelling and Reading." *Learning to Spell: Research, Theory, and Practice Across Languages*. Eds. Charles A. Perfetti, Laurence Rieben, and Michel Foyol. Mahwah, NJ: Lawrence Erlbaum Associates, 1997. 21–38.

Richards, Todd L., Thomas J. Grabowski, Peter Boord, Kevin J. Yagle, Mary K. Askren, Zoe Mestre, Paul Robinson, O. Welker, D. Gulliford, William Nagy, and Virginia W. Berninger. "Contrasting Patterns of Writing-Related DTI Parameters, fMRI Connectivity, and DTI-fMRI Connectivity Correlations in Children with and without Dysgraphia or Dyslexia." *NeuroImage: Clinical* 8 (2015): 408–421.

Saddler, Bruce. *Teacher's Guide to Effective Sentence Writing*. New York: Guilford Press, 2012.

Shaywitz, Sally. *Overcoming Dyslexia*. New York: Vintage Books, 2005.

Stanovich, Keith. "Matthew Effects in Reading: Some Consequences of Individual Differences in the Acquisition of Literacy." *Reading Research Quarterly* 21:4 (Fall 1986): 360–407.

Stone, Gregory O., Mickie Vanhoy, and Guy Van Orden. "Perception Is a Two-Way Street: Feedforward and Feedback Phonology in Visual Word Recognition." *Journal of Memory and Language* 36 (1997): 337–359.

Sumner, Emma, Vincent Connelly, and Anna L. Barnett. "A Review of Dyslexia and Expressive Writing in English." *Writing Development in Children with Hearing Loss, Dyslexia, or Oral Language Problems*. Eds. Barbara Arfe, Julie Dockrell, and Virginia Berninger. Oxford: Oxford University Press, 2014. 188–200.

Sumner, Emma, Vincent Connelly, and Anna L. Barnett. "Children with Dyslexia Are Slow Writers Because They Pause More Often and Not Because They Are Slow at Handwriting Execution." *Reading and Writing: An Interdisciplinary Journal* 26 (2013): 991–1008.

Sumner, Emma, Vincent Connelly, and Anna L. Barnett. "The Influence of Spelling Ability on Vocabulary Choices When Writing for Children with Dyslexia." *Journal of Learning Disabilities* 49:3 (May–June 2016): 293–304.

Ziegler, Johannes, and Ludovic Ferrand. "Orthography Shapes the Perception of Speech: The Consistency Effect in Auditory Word Recognition." *Psychonomic Bulletin & Review* 5 (1998): 683–689.

Ziegler, Johannes, Ludovic Ferrand, and Marie Montant. "Visual Phonology: The Effects of Orthographic Consistency on Different Auditory Word Recognition Tasks." *Memory and Cognition* 32:5 (2004): 732–741.

Index

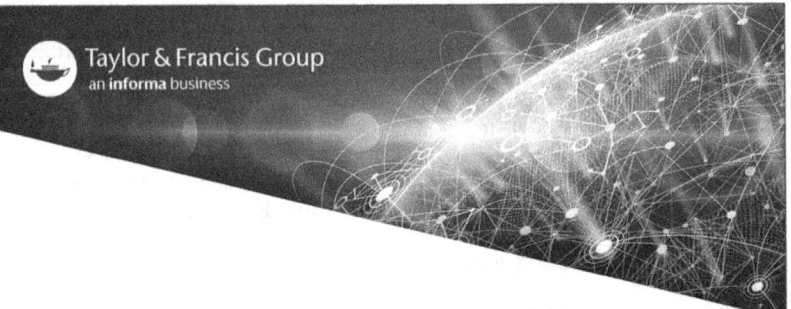
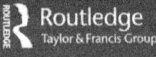
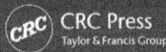